Praise for Heal Thyself

Dr. Pieter De Wet, MD provides a unique insight into the miracle of life and the fact that, in almost every instance, you can personally transform your health with the knowledge and wisdom found in his writings. *Heal Thyself* defines the problems with our current flawed healthcare system, while explaining what illness is and what illness is not. The roles of inner conflicts, toxins, infectious organisms, belief systems, negative emotions, and more, as being the true causes of health challenges are explored in depth. You will develop an understanding of what they are and what you can do to overcome almost any health challenge.

—Frank Jordan, host of "Frank Jordan's
Healthy, Wealthy, and Wise Show"

Dr. Pieter De Wet has written a book that every patient should read in order to gain optimum health. *Heal Thyself* helps even the novice patient understand how most illnesses actually develop and how the patient can take responsibility for their own recovery using safe, effective, noninvasive techniques. Most physicians should be required to read *Heal Thyself*, not only to better understand the true causes of chronic diseases and the safest and most effective tools to resolve those diseases, but also to better understand why the current medical system in the United States is broken and how it can be repaired. I praise Dr. De Wet for his boldness in telling his readers the truth about health and disease, for the clear, understandable way he presents these truths and for the action steps he recommends for patients to start moving toward health.

—William Lee Cowden, MD, MD(H),
chairman of Scientific Advisory Board of IntegraMed Academy,
co-author of *An Alternative Medicine Definitive Guide to Cancer, Cancer Diagnosis: What To Do Next,* and *Longevity, An Alternative Medicine Definitive Guide*

Heal Thyself is an excellent A-Z, what you need to do in order to truly get well naturally. Everything Dr. Pieter De Wet has written is totally true. It should be required reading in every medical school and for every serious patient wanting to get truly well.

—Bruce H. Shelton, MD, MD(H), DiHom FBIH

Heal Thyself

Heal Thyself

Transform Your Life
Transform Your Health

Pieter de Wet, MD

TATE PUBLISHING & Enterprises

Published by Tate Publishing & Enterprises, LLC
127 E. Trade Center Terrace | Mustang, Oklahoma 73064 USA
1.888.361.9473 | www.tatepublishing.com

Tate Publishing is committed to excellence in the publishing industry. The company reflects the philosophy established by the founders, based on Psalm 68:11,
"The Lord gave the word and great was the company of those who published it."

Book design copyright © 2010 by Tate Publishing, LLC. All rights reserved.
Cover and Interior design by Blake Brasor

Published in the United States of America

ISBN: 978-1-61663-672-2
1. Medical, Alternative Medicine
2. Self-help, General
10.04.13

Acknowledgments

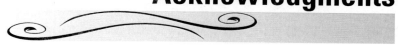

This book is the end product of an almost ten-year odyssey that started because of my realization that in order to be more efficient in my practice of holistic medicine, I needed to be more efficient in educating my patients in regards to what was making them sick and what they could do to get well again. I especially wanted to help them gain knowledge on what they could do for themselves at home, on their own steam, in this era of skyrocketing health care costs and a health care system almost exclusively focused on treating symptoms and not causes. I count myself very fortunate to be in a position to be able to practice medicine based on the holistic model in spite of all the challenges and even heartache that it has brought at times, and I have been able to do so only because of the support of so many, including my family, friends, colleagues, mentors, and the thousands of wonderful and inspiring people that have come to me as patients. I have learned so much from each one of them.

I could not be doing what I am doing in medicine and attempting to find time to write books and teach if it wasn't for the unconditional and loving support of my wife, best friend, and business partner, Cindi. She inspires me every day for so many reasons, including the fact that she has entrusted me with the opportunity to assist her with her health. Her dedication and hard work have helped her overcome a number of debilitating health challenges over the years. She has been an inspiration to so many others because of her own path of health transformation. I am also deeply indebted to the rest of my family—including my seven kids, Kara, Wayne, Morgan, Gabe, Eli,

Sharn, and Keerin, for their love and support; Sharn, in particular, for his dedication in assisting me in my work as a healer, and Keerin for the many hours she spent helping me get this text down in print. I also want to thank my father-in-law, Richard Hickey, for his moral and technical support and for providing a haven in magical San Carlos, Mexico, for me to be able to go into relative seclusion in order to be able to focus on writing; my mother-in-law, Dottie Smith, for helping run our household in order for me and Cindi to do the work that we do to help others; and dear friends, including Ed Johnson, whose editing assistance has been a great help.

I also thank others, including my sister, Renee Brits; friends, including David Goughnour, Billie Garmon, Chris Sebonya, and Julia Schulenberg, N.MD; and staff members of Quantum Healing Institute, including Vanessa Hunter and Carol Pulis for their support and assistance in reviewing text and giving me their input regarding this book. I also deeply appreciate the support of enablers, including Clarence and Corene Schwab, Elizabeth "Dee" Saba, as well as Pierre De Wet, for their moral and financial support over the years that has made all this possible.

I also feel deeply indebted to my mentors in the health care field who have been so instrumental in shaping my perspectives on health care, on what is making us sick as a society and what we can do to help people get back on track. I'll start with Lee Cowden, MD, who has played a huge role in helping me understand so much and has given me the courage to change my path accordingly; Dietrich Klinghardt, MD, PhD, who has helped me gain insight into the different levels at which disease develops and how to assist in healing at these levels of disease entry; Bruce Shelton, MD and Alta Smit, MD, who have both given me a greater understanding on homotoxicology and how we get sick; and Joe Mercola, MD, who has been one of the loudest voices out there calling for reform in health care and has shed a light on those industries that are contributing to the myriad of chronic disease epidemics. He has inspired me to stand up for what is right in health care. I owe a special debt of gratitude to Gilbert Renaud, PhD and David Holt, DO, H.MD from whom

I have learned so much about the principles of Recall Healing, Total Biology, and Germanic New Medicine. These principles explain the root of the root of why we get sick in the first place and how to assist in healing at the very deepest levels. Both chapters on Recall Healing in this book include summaries of what I have learned, especially from these two giants, in the field of Recall Healing and Total Biology. I would also be remiss if I did not mention others that I have been deeply inspired by, including David Hawkins, MD, PhD, who is quoted many times in this book and who has made a big difference as far as helping us understand the whole subject of consciousness; Anthony Robbins, who has influenced me and millions of others around the globe to live more effective and fulfilling lives; Dr. Wayne Dyer, who has been a great inspiration, starting with the very first book of his that I read (*Real Magic*) and continuing with so many of his other books since; Deepak Chopra, MD, who was my original inspiration for renaming my clinic the Quantum Healing Institute after I read his book, *Quantum Healing*, and continued to inspire me with many of his other books and courses since; Larry Dossey, MD, with his brilliant insights into the shifting eras of medicine, especially on the newest era, that of spirit-mind-body medicine, and his work on spiritual healing; and Doug Kaufman and Frank Jordan, who have inspired me to speak out on my beliefs about health care, including the controversial ones, and who have given me opportunities to share my thoughts on their inspirational health care-oriented shows on radio and television.

I also wish to thank Kathy and Pat Jackson for their love and encouragement through the years and their help with keeping my feet to the fire; Ed and Cindy Burson, who have inspired me and my wife, Cindi, to learn the secrets of organic gardening for our own benefit and to encourage others to follow suit in their pursuit of better health; and John and Vicki Yahn for their hours of training and support helping us to start our own radio show, the *Quantum Healing Hour* on XM radio which has given me and my wife an additional forum to connect with others interested in learning about self healing.

I have referred to a number of concepts in the book that have been presented by various authors. The fact that I refer to specific items with which I agree does not mean that I agree with all of any particular author's opinions.

Most importantly, I acknowledge my Creator, the Source of all things, including this book.

•

Table of Contents

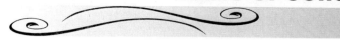

Introduction 15
Part I: The Problem: Our Health in Jeopardy 23
   Catastrophic Meltdown of Health Care in the USA 24
   Limitations of Conventional Medicine 29
   Lifestyle 41
   Toxic Environment 57
   Big Pharma 63
   Selling Sickness 70
   Food Supply in Jeopardy 81
   Is Modern Technology Making Us Sick?. 87
Part II: The Roots of Illness and Pathway to Wellness. 91
   Unresolved Inner Conflicts and the Root Causes of Illness. .92
   The Anatomy of an Illness. 124
   The Five Levels of Healing 139
   Erroneous Belief Systems. 145
   Stress, Negative Emotions, and Your Health 160
   Relationships and Your Health 171
   Spiritual Roots of Illness 180

Part III: The Cure: Your Guide to Miraculous Healing 187

  A Shift in Consciousness 188

  Healing Through Recall 192

  Basic Steps Toward Optimum Health 222

    Step 1: Eat Your Way Back to Health

    Step 2: Alkalinize

    Step 3: Ensure Adequate Water Intake

    Step 4: Exercise

    Step 5: Get Enough Exposure to Sunlight

    Step 6: Get Enough Fresh Air

    Step 7: Get Enough Sleep

    Step 8: Reduce Exposure to Food-Borne and
        Environmental Toxins

    Step 9: Reduce EMF (Electromagnetic Field) Exposure

    Step 10: Detoxify or Die

    Step 11: Heal False Beliefs

    Step 12: See the Humor in Everything

    Step 13: Be at Peace With Loss

    Step 14: Live a Purpose-Driven Life

    Step 15: Heal Your Relationships

    Step 16: Foster an Attitude of Gratitude

    Step 17: Nurture a Direct Relationship With Your Creator

    Step 18: Altruism—In Service of Life and the Living

Twelve-week Action Plan to Manifest Your Miracle 343

Bibliography 369

Resources 373

There are only two ways to live your life. One is as though there are no miracles. The other is as though everything is a miracle.

—Albert Einstein

Miracles happen not in opposition to nature, but in opposition to what we know of nature.

—Arthur C. Clark

Introduction

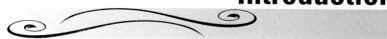

Disease is the brain's best solution to keep the person alive as long as possible; therefore, disease is a survival program.

—Dr. Claude Sabbah

To heal from any illness, it is necessary and sufficient to remove the source of conflict within oneself.

—Dr. Claude Sabbah

Is disease a curse, or is it a solution? As a matter of fact, an even more profound question would be, "Is disease a curse or a blessing?" *Heal Thyself: Transform Your Life, Transform Your Health* is a book designed to shed new light on the way we get sick and shows a more empowering perspective on disease in general. It is more importantly a guidebook on how to dramatically increase the odds of healing from what ails you and how to stay disease-free once healing has taken place. The steps highlighted in this book are so powerful if followed that recovery from even serious health challenges is often the result. This book also will help you create a more empowering framework in which disease can be seen for what it really is: a biological solution and not a curse. In fact, I want to take it further and help readers see that there is nothing random about illness, that it is part of the perfection of creation. If illness is a solution and not a curse, it can ultimately be reframed as a blessing. After reading this book, my hope is that every reader will have a greater appreciation for the miracle of life, the miracle that each one of us is, and the miracle of this extraordinary creation that we are a part of.

It is essential that we look at disease in a totally new way, because the current way is not serving us. The traditional view of illness is that it is a randomly occurring scourge that is at best related to our imperfect makeup and genetic code or our increasingly toxic environment and food supply. Some even attempt to frame it from a religious perspective as punishment from God for our sins. These negative perspectives have formed key beliefs and motivations for the wars that are being fought against illness and that are failing to stem the tide of misery.

We use terms like the "war against cancer," the "war against heart disease," the "war against AIDS," the "war against diabetes," and so on, and have spent billions of dollars in an attempt to find cures with only limited success. It is true that people are living longer, in general, and more specifically with chronic illnesses, such as those listed above, but the incidence of these illnesses and others continues to skyrocket. Ironically, it seems that the more money that we throw at the problem and the more awareness we build through our schools and our media about these diseases, the more common these illnesses become.

Heal Thyself aims to have the reader understand that the idea that we should be fighting against disease, instead of building an awareness of its underlying purpose and resolving it at a deeper level, actually accentuates disease and makes it worse. By understanding the purpose of disease and its root causes, the solutions become readily apparent. As a matter of fact, there is such simplicity to it that my contention is that almost anybody can learn to at least make a start at addressing these causes. They can come up with many of their own solutions with the help of this book and the help of carefully chosen health care professionals, family members, and friends. The purpose of this book is to empower you to embrace the solutions that are there for you, to no longer feel that you are at the mercy of something so huge, devastating, and out of your control that you succumb to the mass consciousness of a particular illness,

therefore allowing yourself to become defeated because of a lack of knowledge.

The first part of this book, "The Problem: Our Health in Jeopardy," delves into the inexorable, worsening epidemics of chronic illness, in spite of the fortunes that are being spent to fight them. This also is in spite of an ever-increasing number of procedures being done and new drugs, which only seem to make us sicker. We discuss in this section who and what is to blame, including the role of conventional medicine, the pharmaceutical industry, and other food and chemical industries. This section will open your eyes to the way we are all blindly being led to the slaughter.

The second part of the book, "The Roots of Illness and Pathway to Wellness," endeavors to help create a deeper understanding of what illness is all about, that illness is a solution and a blessing, not a problem and a curse. As a matter of fact, the first chapter in this part delves right into what I believe to be the most important discovery ever made in medicine: the critical role of inner conflicts as the root cause of all disease and the biological laws that apply. I also discuss the role that belief systems, negative emotions, and relationship challenges play in the development of health problems, and delve into the spiritual roots of illness. In this part, we also discuss the homotoxicology perspective, which understands illness as related to the disruption of the body's defense against the influx of toxins and infectious agents and describes symptoms of illness as evidence of and the expression of these defense mechanisms in action. This part also explains how detrimental it is to suppress symptoms with conventional medical interventions, including pharmaceuticals, in the "battle" to restore one's health, instead of treating the root causes of illness.

The last part of this book, "The Cure: Your Guide to Miraculous Healing," explores a series of solutions to health problems that can be implemented by most people on their own. It lays the groundwork for taking responsibility for initiating the necessary steps for self-healing instead of counting on a flawed health care system. True healing can only be achieved by dealing with health challenges on all

levels, including the physical, mental, emotional, spiritual, social, and environmental levels; in other words, by taking a holistic approach.

My Passion

Ever since I can remember, I wanted to be a doctor. My father, who was a chiropractor, was my first and most influential role model. He was a deeply dedicated and powerful healer, revered as such by thousands of patients who would travel from far and wide to have him lay hands on them to treat their painful conditions. He was very orthodox in his use of chiropractic techniques and yet had a profound impact on his patients beyond what could be explained by the manipulation techniques he employed to treat his patients. His loving spirit and compassionate care touched his patients at deeper levels, giving relief not just to their physical pain, but also to the emotional wounds associated with their ailments.

I knew I wanted to be a healer like my dad at the tender age of four years old and started medical school at age seventeen with the encouragement from my dad. He steered me toward becoming an MD rather than a doctor in his profession so that I would have more freedom to include a wider variety of healing tools than otherwise would have been allowed. It was challenging at times to go through the indoctrination of conventional medical education with its strong aversion to the natural therapies that I had grown up with, but I eventually found my peace with it, realizing that my education in conventional medicine would not be wasted. Conventional medical training gave me a strong foundation in learning how the body worked, in diagnosing disease, and in drug therapy and procedures that I still use and find helpful, especially in emergency situations. On the other hand, I was reminded every day why I could never be at peace using strictly conventional methods to treat chronic or non-life-threatening acute diseases. I saw firsthand day to day how severely skewed the treatments and disease models were that were being used in conventional medicine.

After my residency in family medicine, I stayed on as a faculty

member, participating in the education of medical students and physicians in residency training. During my seven-year-long academic career at The University of Texas Health Science Center in Tyler, Texas, I was given the opportunity and the support to create and lead a new department titled the Center for Nutrition and Preventive Medicine. This allowed me to follow and teach the principles of a more holistic model of care. During my time in academic medicine, I gained an even deeper understanding of the frustrations that so many well-meaning physicians and other health care professionals have in their attempt to provide good health care, frustrations leading from the fact that conventional medicine is so focused on the management of the symptoms of disease instead of the root causes. As a matter of fact, I came to realize that every part and aspect of the system, from the control of insurance companies to the influence of drug companies to the training of physicians to the apathy of the general population and politicians, ensured the marginalization of holistic, or integrative medicine.

Since 1997, I have been in private practice, where I now have the privilege to follow my passion, which is to practice holistic, integrative "wellness" medicine. I am now better able to help people discover the root of their health problems and to assist them back to health or, at a minimum, alleviate suffering by blending together the best of natural and conventional medicine. I am in the privileged position to be able to help people see how their health challenges may actually be blessings and not curses and how people may be able to get back in the driver's seat to steer themselves back to health. My greatest passion is to teach and to be a cheerleader to those who are open to a new, more empowering path and who are willing to take greater responsibility for themselves and their loved ones. My greatest hope is that our medical community, insurance industry, and politicians will support a more empowering approach to health care, an approach that encourages the individual to play a more proactive role in their own health care, and an approach that supports that. If I am able to play even a small role in this awakening, I will be greatly honored.

 Transform Your Health

Time to Take a Quantum Leap

As I write this book, I'm distracted by the expanding financial crisis sweeping like a tsunami around the globe. The United States and other governments are pumping trillions of dollars into their economies in an attempt to stabilize them—dollars that they don't have. Not even the savviest financial experts know exactly what to do at this point to bring sanity back to their financial systems. A cloud of fear and panic is descending over us and stealing our joy and peace of mind. A crises mentality has taken hold as millions of people lose their jobs, their homes, and their sense of security. Not only are people being affected financially, but health wise as well. This global crisis adds to the health challenges that we now face and adds to the vicious cycle of stress, disease, and misery that we see around us. As you will learn in the chapter entitled, "Unresolved Inner Conflicts and the Root Cause of Illness" these types of unresolved conflicts are the main triggers for physical and psychological ailments. This phenomenon is a result of the brain downloading these conflicts to itself and other organs and tissues.

Not only is our financial system broken, but our health care system is broken as well. In fact, our failed health care system is a major contributor to the financial crises we are experiencing. With health care costs increasing at three times the rate of regular inflation, the expenditures on health care have created a huge burden on the government, the industries of the country, and taxpayers alike. One would expect that with all of this money going into health care, we would be experiencing improvements in overall health statistics, decreased pain and suffering, and progress in our battle against chronic disease in general. Unfortunately, this is not the case. As a matter of fact, the majority of us are failing miserably in our battle to get or stay healthy.

So, what are our options? In this book, I will show you not only how to survive these troubling times, but how to thrive. The challenge is to find the silver lining in this dark cloud. Crisis is like a furnace. It can burn you up and destroy you, or it can help you recast

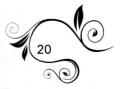

yourself. The primary negative emotion that most people are currently dealing with is fear. Fear of loss, fear that they are not enough, or fear that they don't have what it takes to survive. Even fear that they won't be loved or appreciated or have enough worth, especially by those who look up to them and depend on them. And fear can either serve us by pulling us out of our comfort zones, forcing us to take positive action, or it can paralyze us.

It is in times like this that we realize more than ever that there is no one out there who is going to rescue us. We have to rescue ourselves. Let's face the fact now that in order to survive, we have to change our course dramatically in all realms of our lives, starting with our health. If you lose your health, you have lost your most valuable asset to help you out of this rut. You cannot afford to waste another moment before getting down and dirty and get your health on the right track or make the effort to keep it on the right track. Not only can you conquer this crisis, but you can take advantage of it. Let these challenges strengthen you and help you to become more creative, expanding your vision of what is possible.

Now is the time to make critical decisions like moving forward to reform your lifestyle, to change your eating habits, to start getting regular exercise, and to find ways to support your body in healing itself naturally. This is also the time to strengthen your faith, to conquer negative emotional patterns, and to heal your most valued relationships. There are examples in this book of people who have overcome seemingly insurmountable challenges through following this direction.

In this book, you will learn that suffering is not related to what is happening to you or around you, but is related to how you interpret what is happening. You will learn to focus on what you can control—especially on what you want. This book will help you to crystallize your personal action plan. You will learn how to create an action plan that details exactly what needs to happen to ensure the achievement of your goals.

It is time to take the "quantum leap" and experience your true potential and our potential as a global society.

Part I
The Problem
Our Health in Jeopardy

Health Care USA

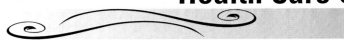

Catastrophic Meltdown

There is no way to be nice about this. There is no point in raising false hopes. There is no treatment or vaccine in sight. There is no miracle breakthrough on the horizon. Medicine as we know it, is dying. It is entering a terminal phase. What began as an acute illness reached the chronic stage about a decade ago, and progression toward death has been remarkably swift and well beyond anything one could have predicted.

—Health Reporter Nick Regush

America with all its ingenuity, entrepreneurship, generosity, and perseverance is facing a catastrophic meltdown of its health care system. This may seem like an extreme statement, but when you review the evidence with me, I believe you will agree. The United States, the richest nation on earth, spends more money per person ($7,681 per person in 2008) on health care by a margin of more than two to one, compared with most other industrialized nations. National health care expenditures in the United States have increased more than eighteen-fold (from $135 billion to $2.5 trillion) since 1970, even though the consumer price index has only increased five-fold. Health care inflation, in other words, is running at more than three times the overall inflation rate in this country, and health care costs have been doubling on average every seven years since 1960. Health care as a percentage of gross domestic product has gone from 5 percent in 1960 to over 16 percent today and at current rates will hit 20 percent by 2016.

Transform Your Life

The question that we need to ask is, *What is all this money buying us?* With politicians promising that even more of our tax dollars will be going into health care, for example, to cover the over forty-seven million people in our country without health insurance, this question needs to be answered urgently. All this expenditure seems counterproductive when you realize that we are over $14 trillion in debt as a nation as of February 2010. This trend of skyrocketing health care costs is predicted to continue unabated unless drastic action is taken by our politicians who up to now have refused to step up to the plate. This is particularly ironic when you realize that the quality of health has been going down sharply over the last three to four decades. For example, the United States used to be ranked No. 1 in terms of life expectancy as recently as thirty years ago and now ranks forty-second in overall life expectancy and thirty-fourth in terms of infant survival.

In America, preventable causes of death continue to rise, along with the incidence of chronic diseases, such as heart disease, cancer, and diabetes, in spite of the almost $2.5 trillion spent on health care per year (expected to rise to about $4 trillion by 2017). The amount of pain and suffering from all manner of chronic illnesses continues to rise, affecting more and more people at younger and younger ages. For instance, obesity and all the health problems associated with it continues to skyrocket, with an estimated 65 percent of adults now considered to be overweight and one-third classified as obese (over 20 percent above ideal body weight). As we age, weight problems become even worse, with an estimated 80 percent of adults over twenty-five years of age being overweight.

Many of our politicians are telling us that the United States has the best health care system in the world, but it is clear for anybody to see how deceptive this statement is. The truth is that we may very well have the best disease care system in the world, a system that extracts ever-increasing rivers of money from consumers and taxpayers with a promise of a quick fix "miracle" solution to every ill. The irony is that there seems to be a reverse correlation between

expenditures on health care and health outcomes. The reasons for this will be explained later.

Another dubious distinction is that the United States leads the world in medical errors and inefficient health care. The most common errors included wrong medications, inaccurate or delayed test results, and improper treatment. Of course, Americans take a lot more drugs for health problems than any other nation, so there is a lot more room for error. I do not want to make it sound like conventional medicine is all bad, because it isn't. There is a lot of good to say about the extraordinary strides that have been made in diagnosis and treatment of acute, as well as chronic illness in this country and around the world. Hundreds of thousands of health care providers toil ceaselessly in an effort to alleviate suffering and often do so successfully. Conventional medicine has a critical role to play in the care of illness today and will in the future, but there is also a lot that is wrong with the treatment paradigm that underpins so much of conventional medicine.

Scary Doctor Facts

1. The number of physicians in the United States is 700,000.
2. Accidental deaths directly related to the actions of physicians per year are around 120,000.
3. Accidental deaths per physician are 0.171.

(Statistics courtesy of US Department of Health and Human Services)

Then think about this:

1. The number of gun owners in the United States is 80 million.
2. The number of accidental gun deaths per year (all age groups) is 1,500.
3. The number of accidental deaths per gun owner is 0.0000188.

(Statistics courtesy of FBI)

Statistical fact: Doctors are approximately 9,200 times more dangerous than gun owners. Conclusion: Guns don't kill people, doctors do. Fact: Not everyone has a gun, but almost everyone has at least one doctor!

What is most shocking is that drugs and doctors are listed as the third-leading cause of death in the United States, responsible for the deaths of around 250,000 people per year. Estimates range from 225,000 to 284,000, and this is in the face of well-recognized underreporting of adverse drug effects by physicians and hospitals. The reported deaths per year include: 106,000 caused by adverse drug effects of drugs that were prescribed inappropriately by physicians, seven thousand medication errors in hospitals alone, twenty thousand other errors in hospitals, eighty thousand hospital-based infections, and twelve thousand unnecessary surgeries.

Conventional medicine, in all likelihood, is the leading cause of death if you take into account that the statistics listed above are mostly derived from studies in hospitalized patients and the fact that autopsies are rarely done on chronically ill patients who die at home. Add to this the fact that conventional medicine almost never confronts the root cause of an illness (only the symptoms) and that medications always add to the toxic load already affecting the body, blowing out those defense mechanisms meant to protect us, and you can understand the conclusion that conventional medicine may be the leading cause of death.

Obviously, the severe dysfunction in our health care system does not just apply to death rates, but is also correlated with a massive burden of pain and suffering and disability among our population. Drug-related adverse effects have been estimated to cost more than $136 billion per year in the United States, which puts it ahead of the total cost of cardiovascular care or diabetes care in this country.

It is estimated that one out of every six (18 percent) American adults of working age were so disabled because of health problems in 2006 that they were unable to work. This is up from 15 percent in 2004. In this same time period, the sales of pharmaceuticals have continued to skyrocket.

The take-home message is that drugs do not prevent or cure anything and are mainly focused on creating pseudo health, which means you feel better for a while because your symptoms are being treated, but the cause has not been addressed. This is what makes conventional medicine so dangerous.

Our health care system is being crushed under the weight of massively growing health care expenditures, with nothing but more death, disease, and dysfunction to show for it. The good news is that the death of symptom-based medicine will lead to a mass reduction in the massive corrupting influence that Big Pharma holds over our society and our political system. What we do *not* need in order to address this problem is:

1. Greater access to more and more drugs, with the government paying a bigger and bigger portion.
2. More stringent drug treatment protocols as part of so-called standardized medicine, or what I call "cookie-cutter medicine" or "one-size-fits-all medicine," with physicians held over a barrel if they don't comply.
3. Patients being penalized if they refuse to take these disease-promoting drugs, especially the ones that are supposed to prevent disease.
4. More and more vaccines for more and more infectious diseases.
5. Government-run socialized medicine with government bureaucrats telling you which doctors you can see and what kind of medicine is allowed to be used.

Unfortunately, this is what the majority of our politicians and the leaders of our health care system are recommending. This will only make matters far worse than they already are because of the simple fact that more government intervention, more drugs, or more than the already astronomical number of vaccines are not the answer; these things are a huge part of the problem.

What we do need is a dramatic shift in our overall philosophy and approach to taking care of health challenges.

Limitations of Conventional Medicine

Who Is to Blame for the Growing Health Care Crisis in America?

There is a growing epidemic of chronic illness in this country in spite of the fortunes being spent on health care. Out of the top ten leading causes of death, nine are due to preventable diseases. Over 650,000 people die every year from coronary artery disease, and over 550,000 die from cancer. The incidence of cancer has increased from approximately one in a hundred in 1900 to one in two today. Once a person is diagnosed with cancer, the chance of dying has not significantly changed in the last one hundred years. What has changed is the skyrocketing incidence of the diagnosis. This is in spite of the fact that well over $200 billion have been spent on fighting the "war on cancer" since it was declared by President Richard Nixon in 1971.

Leading causes of death in the United States:

1. Heart disease—651,696
2. Cancer—559,228
3. Stroke—143,449
4. Chronic lower respiratory disease—130,896
5. Unintentional injury—116,669
6. Diabetes mellitus—75,118
7. Alzheimer's disease—71,598
8. Influenza and pneumonia—62,734
9. Nephritis—43,742

Transform Your Health

10. Septicemia—33,831

Source: CDC, 2005.

The incidence of type 2 diabetes increased by over 50 percent from 1995 to 2005 and has doubled over the past twenty-five years, affecting people at younger and younger ages, with the most rapid increases in the age group from birth to forty-four years of age (0.8 per hundred in 1995 to 1.4 per hundred in 2005). As a matter of fact, out of this group, teenagers are seeing the fastest growth in a disease that until twenty-five years ago rarely occurred in adults under forty-four years of age. Even in the youngest members in our community, things are going from bad to worse, with the incidence of autism, for example, having increased a staggering 1,200 percent in the last fifteen years, and conditions such as ADHD (attention deficit hyperactivity disorder) and teenage depression are skyrocketing.

In addition, more people are suffering from hypertension, chronic fatigue, chronic arthritis, chronic low back pain, and headaches than ever before. More kids are suffering from ADHD, depression, autism, and other psychiatric illnesses than ever before. One in six kids now has a severe learning disorder. More and more women are suffering from PMS, osteoporosis, hot flashes, night sweats, sexual dysfunction, and so on. An increasing segment of the male population is suffering from enlarged prostates, enlarged breasts, and impotence. More and more people are suffering from severe reflux disease, poor digestion, constipation, and irritable bowel disease.

Almost everywhere you turn, it becomes readily apparent that the incidence of a vast array of chronic illnesses is increasing, not just in our adult population but in our children and teenagers as well. The only conclusion that we can draw is that in spite of billions of dollars spent on research into drug and other conventional therapies and in spite of trillions of dollars spent on health care, not only are we not gaining ground, we are actually losing ground.

For many of you, these statistics come as a great shock because of the media's failure to report the facts. Information on the most egregious threats to our existence is being swept under the rug regularly,

Transform Your Life

while far lesser threats are gaining headlines. Every little outbreak of food-borne illness will dominate media coverage for days or weeks even though very few people may die, whereas the staggering death rates from preventable diseases, such as heart disease and cancer, and death rates from medical mistakes are hardly ever mentioned. This conspiracy of silence is a direct result of special interest groups tied up in profiteering from drug sales, medical services, and other medical technologies, and the sway that they hold over the media and our politics.

The consequences of this conspiracy are devastating in so many ways. For example, it is estimated that 1.2 million people per year are declaring bankruptcy as a direct result of unexpected out-of-pocket medical costs. Small and large businesses are finding it harder and harder to cover their employees with medical insurance. Even some of the owners are going without. With the growing worldwide financial crisis, our astronomical and growing national debt, and with the baby boomer generation retiring in droves over the next twenty or so years, our present health care infrastructure will be unable to handle the load.

Is Conventional Medicine to Blame?

I do not believe for a moment that the average physician in America has any intention to harm their patients. In fact, the vast majority of physicians are dedicated servants doing their best to meet the medical needs of their patients in spite of daunting obstacles, such as lack of time, skyrocketing costs, more and more paperwork, greater patient dissatisfaction, and the threat of malpractice suits. In addition, many of them are working harder and harder for less and less pay. Please don't misunderstand; medicine is still one of the best-paid professions in the country, but it is still disconcerting for physicians to see their paychecks shrinking and with politicians threatening them with even more cuts in reimbursement through programs like Medicare and Medicaid. The sad thing is that over a third of physicians now say that they would not enter the profession

were they to do it all over again, and less than a third of physicians are happy with the direction medicine is going in. This is especially true for the primary care specialties such as internal medicine, family medicine, and pediatrics.

Most physicians are not aware of all the dire statistics (mentioned before) that stand as an indictment against traditional medicine. In all fairness, doctors themselves are not to blame for all of this except in the sense that most of them live in willful ignorance. How else can you explain their lack of action as a group against medical organizations, pharmaceutical companies, and insurance companies that embody this fatally flawed health care paradigm that is contributing to this massive epidemic of chronic disease that is so apparent for anyone to see?

A Fatally Flawed Paradigm

America leads the world in terms of health care infrastructure. We have the best hospitals in the world in terms of having the best and most abundantly available equipment, the best-trained physicians and support staff, and the latest and best drugs to work with. Our health care system is unparalleled in its ability to image, test, diagnose, and treat, yet seemingly nearly unable to make a dent in the incidence and progression of chronic illnesses. We are becoming sicker and sicker as a nation.

The problem is a fatally flawed paradigm with its entire focus on the wrong end of the problem. We are becoming ever more efficient at controlling the symptoms of disease with little attention being paid to the root causes. Almost the entire focus of conventional medicine, with all its wonderful drugs and mechanical interventions, is on minimizing and suppressing symptoms as efficiently as possible. As a matter of fact, when they are successful at treating these symptoms they call it victory over chronic disease even though the disease itself persists and usually ends up getting worse over time.

When it comes to root causes, the chronic disease epidemic is

explained away in large part due to genetic abnormalities. In order to accept this explanation as the main cause of disease, we also have to accept that our genes have suddenly mutated. Based on the dramatic rise in the incidence of chronic illnesses of almost all types at younger and younger ages; this explanation simply does not hold up to scrutiny.

In addition to genetics, poor lifestyle choices and other factors, such as environmental toxicity, also get blamed as a significant contributor, but hardly ever get addressed by conventional health care providers, except for the occasional abbreviated admonition to do something in particular like stop smoking, eat less, exercise more, or reduce stress. These factors certainly do play very important roles in the development of disease, but there is far more to it than this.

As mentioned before, most physicians simply don't have time, knowledge, or the opportunity to really educate or support themselves or their patients on this front. Physicians get almost nonstop education on drug therapies starting from the time they walk into medical school. A huge portion of this education and incentive to prescribe drugs comes directly from the drug industry in the form of drug reps hovering around physicians' offices on a daily basis encouraging (some call it bribing) physicians with free meals, free entertainment, free drug samples, and other free goodies.

Then there is also the drug industry's paid surrogates giving lectures accompanied by fine dining in the best restaurants around and the drug company sponsorship of medical conferences and medical school activities. In order to show their gratitude, physicians return the favor by prescribing the drugs produced by these drug companies.

In contrast, physicians receive almost no training on nutrition and true preventive medicine. Virtually the only training in preventive medicine that physicians get during or after medical school is on screening for disease and immunizations.

Why is it important to track down and treat causes rather than just simply treat the symptoms? What's wrong with just blowing out symptoms that make us uncomfortable and miserable? Is it pos-

sible that by interfering with symptoms, we are actually affecting the body's ability to defend itself? Is it possible that our bodies were created in such a way that they can actually heal themselves, given the right circumstances?

I believe it is critical to track down and treat the root causes of illness because simply treating symptoms dramatically escalates disease progression. It is absolutely true that when we treat symptoms, we impair the body's ability to defend and protect itself.

And God said:

> Let us make man in our image, after our likeness.
>
> Genesis 1:26

Each one of us inhabits a miraculous body that under the right circumstances and given the right support can heal itself in extraordinary ways. The body has the innate ability to heal itself when given the space to do so by eliminating the factors that impede healing, like toxicity, nutrient deficiencies, toxic emotions, and, most importantly, unresolved conflicts.

> Beloved, I wish above all things that thou mayest prosper and be in health, even as thy soul prospereth.
>
> 3 John 1:2

> For I will restore health unto thee, and I will heal thee of thy wounds, saith the LORD.
>
> Jeremiah 30:17

When we came into this world, we were each gifted with an extraordinary body, which by adulthood contains around 100 trillion cells, all somehow connected, functioning in concert with each other every split second of every day. This not only allows us to survive and thrive in physical form, but to experience this miraculous universe around us in incredible ways, enabling us to experience love, joy, and inner peace on the one hand, and pain and suffering on the other. Most of us abhor pain and suffering until we realize their spiritual purpose, which is to help us become more aware of who we are and what

our true potential is. Pain and suffering also coax us to learn how to feed and nurture our bodies back to health, not just in the physical realm, but also in the emotional, mental, social, and spiritual realms. Struggle is an integral and growth-promoting part of life starting at the very beginning, when we first make our appearance into this world. The suffering entailed in the birth process itself, for mother and child alike, is almost instantly transformed at birth into ecstasy and exhilaration as the child takes its first breath, thereby saving its own life, and then falls into its mother's loving embrace.

Treating Symptoms Is the Problem

So again, why not just treat symptoms? That's simple. Aside from the fact that treating symptoms doesn't treat the cause, our health care system has a vested interest in our getting and staying ill because fortunes are being made on the backs of the sick in our country. Our megalithic health care system would literally fall apart overnight and profits would disappear if we suddenly started treating disease at its root instead of just treating symptoms. And yes, it would be catastrophic to the health care industry if the average person suddenly figured out one day that self-healing is not only possible, but can be relatively simple (especially in the early stages of disease).

Treating the cause also would devastate other industries, such as our major food and agricultural corporations that have a mega-billion-dollar interest in our continuing to eat the same disease-promoting diet that we are eating now. Our government even subsidizes, to the tune of around $25 billion per year, the farmers that specifically grow the produce that is at the root of the problem, including wheat, corn, soy, rice, and even cotton. Cotton is very heavily sprayed with pesticides and herbicides, which end up in our clothes, and then get absorbed through our skin. In addition, many processed foods are made from cottonseed oil, so we become poisoned from cotton that way. If a person lives in an area near cotton fields, the pesticides and herbicides that are sprayed on the cotton field, when there are only

seven-mile-per-hour winds, will travel twenty-five miles in the air. The only solutions are to avoid breathing or to move.

These subsidies ensure that the most toxic foods that we consume are also the cheapest to manufacture. Certain industries, such as the fast food industry, can sell food very inexpensively because most ingredients are so cheap, including wheat, soy, partially hydrogenated soy oil used in frying foods, high-fructose corn syrup in the soft drinks, and so forth. Corn and soy are also the two crops that are most commonly genetically engineered (Frankenfoods).

School lunch programs around the country also become dumping grounds for these cheap subsidized foods. In other words, our schools are literally sponsoring the indoctrination of our children to become fast food consumers. The parents of those school-aged children were children themselves just a generation ago, and because of their indoctrination, they are feeding their kids and themselves the same foods at home. This is even more pronounced in the inner cities where fresh produce is almost impossible to find and where liquor stores and gas stations are the only game in town and only sell junk foods with these same subsidized ingredients.

Even the diet industry is in the game because of its use of subsidized ingredients such as maltodextrin, which is derived from corn. They hide behind junk science that has supported the sale of so-called "low-fat foods" filled with refined grain and other grain byproducts with the promise that these so-called "low-fat foods" would help you to lose weight. Instead, they seem to be having the opposite effect.

How Is Symptom Management a "Problem"?

Symptoms occur as a direct result and a clear reflection of the body's attempt to protect itself against the invasion of toxins and infectious agents through the layers of protection that each one of us was created with. When symptoms become the target for treatment and are effectively suppressed, not only does it not lead to cure, it actually masks further worsening of the underlying disease process and often accelerates the invasion of toxins and microbes into the body, progressively affecting deeper layers of the body and adversely affecting even the emotional sphere of our being.

Making the Case Against Aggressive Pain Management

In conventional medicine, there is a large emphasis on pain suppression and even entire specialties focused almost exclusively on managing pain. Isn't that the whole purpose of medicine, to alleviate pain and suffering? This sounds like a noble goal, to allow people to live without pain, but think about it carefully. We have to ask ourselves if pain has a purpose.

Pain is a messenger that is attempting to alert you to an underlying problem. It doesn't make a whole lot of sense just to kill the messenger so you can pretend there is no underlying problem. In other words, you shouldn't suppress pain and ignore its cause. Instead, you might attempt to discover its source. When you suppress pain with the wonderful painkillers available to us, you're again suppressing the body's natural defense mechanisms that are attempting to protect you and are inviting side effects. Depending on the type of drugs used in pain management, these side effects may include heartburn, gut irritability, constipation, fatigue, and depression and may adversely affect other organ functions, such as the liver and kidneys.

It is estimated that acetaminophen (i.e., Tylenol) and nonsteroidal anti-inflammatory drugs (NSAIDs), such as ibuprofen (i.e., Advil or Motrin), are responsible for thirty thousand deaths per year in the United States and for over two hundred thousand hospitalizations. Acetaminophen can cause liver failure (56,000 cases per year in the United States, according to a July 2009 FDA report) and even serious kidney damage, and NSAIDs can cause stomach bleeding and kidney failure, as well as contribute to the marked rise in incidence of congestive heart failure (CHF) and diverticular disease of the large bowel. The use of NSAIDs in people suffering from heart disease increases the risk of CHF by more than tenfold and by more than 60 percent in people without heart disease. (Ref: Archives of Internal Medicine—June 2000; 160: 777–786)

The treatment of reflux/heartburn is another good example of the harm caused by treating symptoms instead of causes. Drugs for heartburn rank as one of the top two most profitable drug categories worldwide. One drug in particular, esomeprazole (Nexium), has been one of the top five best-selling drugs for more than five years with current sales above $5 billion per year worldwide. Most people think that when they have heartburn, it must be due to excess acid in the stomach; however, the symptom usually reflects irritation of the lower part of the esophagus. Most cases of reflux simply have nothing to do with excessive stomach acid production. They have to do with the fact that digestion is not working properly and that food becomes static in the stomach and then after hours will tend to reflux into the esophagus, causing irritation and the symptom of heartburn. What has been discovered is that about 90 percent of people with heartburn actually do not have excessive acid production, but may be making too little acid, causing inefficient and sluggish digestion, increasing the likelihood of reflux occurring.

Why do the drugs work to relieve symptoms then? These drugs are very effective at suppressing acid production to the point where minimal amounts of acid are produced, thereby relieving symptoms. If reflux occurs but very little acid is present in the stomach, there is less irritation to the esophagus, thereby relieving heartburn.

Transform Your Life

What is the downside then? There is a reason we were created to produce acid in our stomachs. With no acid present, digestion, of proteins especially, becomes greatly impaired. The stomach is also unable to sterilize food without high acid levels, leading to more gastrointestinal infections than would otherwise occur. So when you take a drug to shut off acid production, you may be causing other problems as you control the one bothersome symptom of heartburn.

Let's look at what the symptom of heartburn is attempting to tell us. If it is not too much acid in the stomach causing the symptom, then what is it? In the natural medical community, the most common culprit found to contribute to heartburn is food sensitivities. The second most common factor is the inadequate production of stomach acid and enzymes, leading to difficulty digesting food properly. Emotions also play a key role, with worry being a frequent companion to heartburn.

A much more sensible approach, therefore, would be to listen to the body's defense mechanism (heartburn) and support the body's healing by identifying and eliminating the foods you are sensitive to and by ensuring an adequate supply of stomach acid and enzymes for digestion. This can be accomplished by either supporting the body's own production or by taking supplements containing these essential factors. In addition, miraculous healing often occurs when the underlying conflict and the associated emotions are tracked down and resolved or reframed.

Stopping acid production with pharmaceuticals inevitably leads to additional problems such as protein malnutrition, deficiency of key nutrients such as vitamin B12 and a much greater propensity for obesity. Suppressing stomach acid affects protein digestion but not the digestion of simple or processed complex carbohydrates. As a matter of fact, carbohydrate cravings tend to increase as a result of protein and nutrient deficiencies leading to an increased risk of obesity.

Another effect of suppressing acid production is that the stomach cannot sterilize food that is eaten. Normally a stomach kills off bacteria and parasites that do not belong in your body. But when

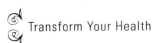

there's no, or very little acid being produced, there is no way for that food to be sterilized. This leads to contamination of the normally sterile small bowel with bacteria and other organisms that shouldn't be there.

For example, if a bacterium like Helicobacter pylori invades the lining of the stomach, it can contribute to the formation of stomach ulcers. It is now generally accepted in the conventional medical community that this organism is the cause of the vast majority of cases of stomach ulcers.

It took a very long time (fifteen years) for conventional medicine to accept the premise that stomach ulcers were caused by an infectious disease. In fact, the physicians who discovered this link, Dr. Barry Marshall and Dr. Robert Warren, had to run the gauntlet of ridicule throughout the medical community around the world, even after one of them infected himself with bacteria and developed an ulcer to prove this link to them.

Things only changed when the pharmaceutical industry took an interest because of the fortunes that could be made if they discovered an antibiotic that could treat this infection effectively and therefore could be used to treat stomach ulcers. This is exactly what happened. All of a sudden, almost overnight, most physicians in the world learned about this new treatment and this new theory on the cause of stomach ulcers. Ironically, today it is deemed malpractice for a physician to treat an ulcer without antibiotics unless he can clearly prove the organism is not present.

There is a great price to pay when you treat symptoms and not causes, including further inhibition of your normal healing response. When you suppress a symptom, you literally turn off the defense mechanism that that symptom is highlighting or pointing to. Pain is always a messenger that needs to be heeded. The body needs to be listened to so that we can allow the body to heal by supporting its defenses—for example, by assisting the body to detoxify itself—which may include supplying essential nutrients and identifying and clearing negative emotions and unresolved conflicts that are interfering with the body's natural healing mechanisms.

Transform Your Life

Lifestyle

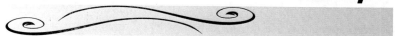

Do our lifestyles contribute to this epidemic of chronic illness? The answer is an unequivocal "yes." Our lifestyle choices, including diet, physical activity levels, substance abuse, and whether or not we get enough sleep have considerable impact on our health. My aim in this chapter is to review some of the most critical mistakes that many of us are making with our lifestyle choices that contribute to our tendency toward ill health. Poor lifestyle choices contribute to the toxic load or what I call the bioload that each one of us carries within our body. By itself this bioload is an important health predictor but even more so when paired with unresolved inner conflicts.

The body's propensity to become poisoned depends not just on the amount of toxin coming into the body but also on the function of individual organ systems, which, in turn, depend heavily on the presence or absence of unresolved inner conflicts.

Diet

Our diets have a huge impact on our overall health status. In so many ways, we are learning that "we are what we eat." It's important that we look more closely at what we are ingesting and whether it promotes health or disease.

It is amazing that a lot of what we have learned about healthy eating over the last thirty to forty years might have been totally wrong. As a matter of fact, there is ample evidence of the harm that has been done through recommendations such as those repre-

sented on the food pyramid, which was first published in 1992. It was designed by a team of top nutritionists sponsored by the United States Department of Agriculture (USDA) but ended up being watered down and altered by the Secretary of Agriculture at the time under apparent pressure from food industry lobbyists attempting to ensure that the food pyramid would not have any negative impact on their industries.

That symbol of healthy eating has been called more and more into question. As a matter of fact, just very recently the whole food pyramid was modified to reflect some of the changes in thinking. Sadly, the new food pyramid, published in 2005, still does relatively little to encourage people to avoid the most harmful foods; for example, those containing processed grains, sugars, artificial sweeteners, partially hydrogenated fats, or GMO (genetically modified organisms) foods. Sadly, again, this is primarily due to the fact that a lot of these recommendations are made based on political expediencies and political interests rather than human health interests.

Partially Hydrogenated Fats

Let's look at a travesty perpetrated decades ago, which is the recommendations made that margarine was somehow better for us than butter. At the time, there were huge special interests pushing the manufacturing of these new products that brought in billions of dollars of profit. We later found out that margarine, which is mostly made up of partially hydrogenated fats, is actually one of the worst poisons that we can consume. It also may be responsible for a large part of the tremendous increase in the incidence of coronary artery disease and cancer in this country.

Trans fats are formed when plant oils are chemically altered to turn them into solids at room temperature, thereby altering their structure in such a way that when incorporated into cell membranes and other structures in the cell, they cause cell dysfunction. For example, cell membranes become very rigid, affecting the absorption of nutrients into the cell, the excretion of toxins out of the cell, and the function of hormone receptors on the cell membrane. Trans

Transform Your Life

fats also have been linked to the dramatic increase in the incidence of coronary artery disease and the hardening of arteries in general, called atherosclerosis. They also have been linked to the dramatic increase in the incidence of cancer and a myriad of other health problems. Trans fats were introduced into our food supply on a large scale starting in the 1950s, which correlates with some of the most dramatic increases in the incidence of serious chronic illnesses in our society today.

Trans fats have become a very popular component of the vast majority of processed foods because of the fact that they dramatically increase the shelf life of food products. This is especially true for those designed to be kept at room temperature.

Artificial Sweeteners

Another group of culprits that came into play a few decades ago were artificial sweeteners, preservatives and artificial flavor, and food texture enhancers. This industry and others made artificial chemicals used in food as ingredients either to maintain or increase shelf life as preservatives or to enhance flavor or texture in order to make artificial food more palatable. In many cases, these chemicals have an addictive effect. More and more evidence is accumulating that not only do these artificial sweeteners and other chemicals fail to help protect us against, for example, obesity, but they might actually make the problem worse because they actually stimulate appetite. There is research that shows that people who consume foods with artificial sweeteners in them do not lose any more weight than people eating foods with regular sugar in them. Many scientists feel very strongly that sugar substitutes, such as aspartame (NutraSweet and Equal), saccharin (Sweet'N Low), and sucralose (Splenda), have negative health effects that far outweigh any benefits a person might gain, such as decreasing caloric intake. For example, aspartame may contribute to symptoms such as headaches, dizziness, irritable bowel, chronic pain (as in fibromyalgia), altered brain function (brain fog), behavioral problems (especially in children), menstrual disorders, and even weakness that can be associated with multiple sclerosis.

These symptoms often disappear almost immediately when this chemical is eliminated from the diet.

There have been very few human studies published on the safety of the artificial sweeteners listed above. In spite of the fact that the FDA has been inundated with consumer complaints, there are also no ongoing studies to evaluate their potential long-term adverse effects.

Splenda is the most recent major addition to the sugar substitute market with a huge question mark regarding its safety in humans. Animal research studies have shown it to cause many adverse effects, including reductions in growth rate in young animals, decreased fetal body weight, suppression of red blood cell counts, enlargement of the liver and kidneys, and suppression of thymus gland function, which controls the immune system. This is just a partial list of the findings in these animal studies. In addition, chemical essays of commercially available sucralose have shown that it contains small amounts of very dangerous substances such as arsenic, lead, and even pesticides.

The addictive potential of artificial sweeteners also is becoming a huge problem and has been compared to other addictions such as nicotine and even cocaine. Thousands of people have reported experiencing severe cravings and withdrawal symptoms when attempting to stop the intake of these products. The difference between artificial sweeteners and other addictive substances mentioned is that products with artificial sweeteners are socially acceptable, freely available, and inexpensive. Cocaine, on the other hand, is illegal, extremely expensive, and hard to come by.

Refined Carbohydrates

It also is becoming abundantly clear that our tremendous emphasis on grains and starches is having catastrophic consequences to our health. Grains are historically a relatively recent addition to our diets. It is only within the last few thousand years, when man started settling down in stable communities that grains came to the forefront. Because of their relative durability and the fact that they

could be stored through the winter, they became the mainstay of the human diet in large parts of the world.

Grains in their unprocessed form, when eaten relatively fresh, can be beneficial but are not critical for human survival. On the other hand, highly processed grains (refined carbohydrates), and simple sugars are in large part responsible for the epidemics of chronic disease in industrialized societies and third-world countries supported by the industrialized world through billions of dollars worth of food donations.

When grain is processed and refined into flour it loses most of its nutrient value except for the calories from starches. Additionally, refined grains are usually bleached to make them white in color. The bleaching process adds to the toxicity of these foods.

Another growing concern is the genetic modification of grains such as corn, as well as other produce, like soy and even certain vegetables and fruits. The goal of genetic modification is to make these plants more resistant to pests and to increase yields in order to expand profitability. Unfortunately, we are all paying a great price for this convenience and at the same time expanding the profits of a handful of very powerful companies.

One of the consequences of genetically modified (GMO) foods is a dramatic increase in the incidence of food sensitivities leading to damage of the intestinal lining. This situation contributes to a myriad of health challenges. Some of these health challenges include irritable bowel syndrome, chronic fatigue, reflux, obesity, and so on. Corn is one example of a grain causing a lot of problems. Almost 100 percent of corn consumed in the US is genetically modified. There is an endless array of food products and even cosmetics that contain corn or corn byproducts such as cornstarch, corn oil, high-fructose corn syrup, dextrose, and maltodextrin. Even many of the supplements and drugs you buy in the local grocery store, pharmacy, or health food store contain corn byproducts or are made from corn. For example, an estimated 99 percent of vitamin C on the market is corn-derived. This can contribute to abnormal sugar metabolism and food sensitivities.

Another consequence is a dramatic increase in the levels of certain toxins (mycotoxins) associated with grains in general, and possibly even more so with wheat and GMO corn, especially those stored in silos for significant periods of time. This does not seem to be a problem with grains such as buckwheat, quinoa, or spelt because they are grown on a much smaller scale and are very seldom stored for more than a few days before processing. Mycotoxins are toxins produced by fungus that grow on stored grains and are known to cause damage to brain cells, the immune system, the liver, and blood vessels and can contribute to a host of serious illnesses, including heart disease, cancer, diabetes, and many others. Our high intake of grains in general, especially refined grains, has contributed greatly to the epidemic of diseases associated with hyperinsulinemia and insulin resistance, including obesity, diabetes, hypertension, high cholesterol, heart disease, cancer, and many more. Grains are made up mostly of starch, especially refined grains (because the fiber is removed), which is rapidly converted into simple sugars in the stomach, leading to a surge of sugar in the bloodstream, necessitating the release of increased amounts of insulin. These levels of sugar are high enough to kill the average cell in the body. The liver has an extraordinary ability to avert this catastrophe by rapidly converting the sugar into fat and cholesterol. These are typically transported from the liver to other tissues such as fat tissue and, unfortunately, even blood vessels. Some of the fat stays behind in the liver often causing fatty liver. This can eventually lead to liver dysfunction. Other health problems including tooth decay occur with increased consumption of grains. According to the studies of Weston Price and Francis Pottenger, those populations around the world that have never eaten grains have much better dental health and overall physical health, compared with those that have. So, next time you decide to treat yourself to a sandwich made of refined, bleached grain derived flour, realize that you may just as well have eaten a candy bar and gotten the same result!

Simple Sugars

The average American today consumes more than 175 pounds of simple sugars per year, compared with less than one pound per year two hundred years ago and less than two pounds per year one hundred years ago. This is in addition to the truckload of refined grains consumed. It is hard to comprehend how we manage to consume this amount of sugar until we look at examples, such as the amount of sugar contained in one can of a regular soft drink. One eight-ounce soft drink may contain the equivalent of approximately ten teaspoons of sugar. "Supersize that" in a fast food drive-thru, and you have doubled or tripled that amount. Add to that the simple sugars used to flavor everything from bread to canned vegetables, and you begin to get the picture. Throw in a few candy bars and some dessert, and you're over the top. This is how people in America are averaging around a half a pound of sugar a day.

Another disturbing fact is that over sixty-two pounds of this sugar consumed consists of high-fructose corn syrup alone. The corn industry in America is heavily subsidized because of the fact that biofuels are made from corn, leading to an abundance of very inexpensive high-fructose corn syrup, which is a byproduct of this manufacturing process. High-fructose corn syrup is even more harmful to the human body than the simple sugar called sucrose derived from sugar cane and beets, which is a lot more expensive than high-fructose corn syrup by the way. This is because of the high incidence of food sensitivity to corn and corn byproducts and the fact that fructose increases insulin production and resistance even more than sucrose and is more addictive.

I have already explained the damaging effects of starches as they get converted into sugar in the stomach. Simple sugars are even more problematic because they move almost unimpeded into the bloodstream from the intestinal tract with only minimal digestion being necessary, leading to very rapid spikes in insulin production, which moves the sugar out of the bloodstream into the cells. Simple sugars contribute to the same health challenges mentioned in the refined carbohydrate section.

Animal Proteins

Animal proteins can be part of a healthy diet, but unfortunately, once again, modern agricultural practices are contributing to the onslaught of disease in our society. Animals like cattle, chickens, turkeys, and pigs are kept in confined spaces in order to minimize calories used for physical exertion and to ensure that as many calories as possible go into growth and fattening of those animals destined for slaughter. The same procedures apply to those animals used for dairy and egg production in order to maximize yield. They are fed high-grain diets, especially with genetically modified and mycotoxin-contaminated corn, instead of their natural diets, such as grass for cattle and seeds and insects for chickens and turkeys. This affects these animals in many adverse ways, which have serious consequences to us when we consume products derived from them. This includes severe depletion of omega-3 fatty acid and conjugated linolenic acid levels and increases in omega-6 fatty acids, not just in the animals themselves but also in those that consume them or their byproducts. This leads to increased inflammation, suppressed immune systems, and all kinds of other negative consequences to those consuming these foods.

Because of their propensity for infections due to their weak immune systems, these animals are often given loads of antibiotics and antiparasitic drugs, which are then consumed by us when we eat these animal products. This is one of the reasons why we are seeing more and more antibiotic-resistant bacteria, or "super bugs," affecting humans and animals and adding to the prospect of germ-based epidemics that we may have to deal with in the future.

Hormones, such as growth hormones, are being used more and more often to speed the growth and increase the size of these animals and to increase milk production in cows. Once again, these hormones enter our bodies, contributing to many health problems.

Processed meats add another layer of toxicity to our diets because of the toxic preservatives that are used.

Acid-Alkaline Imbalance

It is critical to point out that most disease at a foundational level is associated with acid-alkaline imbalance and most diseases are directly related to the over-acidification of blood, lymph fluids, and the intercellular matrix, which leads to over-acidification of the cells. Most bodily functions involving the production of energy at a cellular level are acidifying by nature. One exception involves ammonia production, which is an alkalinizing toxin, as are certain diets that are wrong for one's metabolic type. Excessive alkalinity is usually harder to treat than excessive acidity. Excessive alkalinity represents about 10 percent of the chronically ill patients that I see in my clinic. The vast majority of the rest suffer from excessive acidity. Acid or alkaline byproducts that accumulate in the blood and the tissues of the body inhibit the optimal functioning of the cells and organs of the body, eventually leading to the breakdown of cells.

Major factors contributing greatly to acid-alkaline imbalances:

1. Poor diet, as described earlier in this chapter.
2. Insufficient enzymes for digestion.
3. Inadequate water intake and the consumption of inadequately alkalinized water.
4. Environmental pollution.
5. Lack of exercise.
6. Increased emotional stress and unresolved conflicts.
7. Consumption of food allergens.

Weight Gain

Body fat plays a critical role in maintaining an alkaline pH in the blood and in the tissues, which are critical for the maintenance of life. Body fat acts as a buffer by absorbing and storing acids that the body is unsuccessful at eliminating. This leads to a progressive slowdown of metabolism. Therefore, the tendency is for progressive weight gain as long as the acid problem persists with a myriad

of associated health problems linked to weight gain occurring over time. By the way, you should be eternally grateful for this mechanism, because without it, your body would be awash with acid, literally making life impossible to maintain. As a matter of fact, underweight people faced with excess acid in their system, who are unable to gain weight, are often worse off (health wise) than those who do gain weight.

The failure to address the problem of over-acidity may be the most important reason why even the most aggressive weight loss programs don't work over the long-term. Over 98 percent of people initially successful in losing weight gain all of it and more back within five years.

Infections also are related to acidity.

Excess acidity directly impairs your immune system and promotes the growth of a wide variety of organisms in affected tissues. These include fungus, yeast, bacteria, viruses, and parasites. The more acid in the tissue or blood, the lower the amount of oxygen present and the higher the number of pathogenic organisms. These organisms, in turn, often create additional toxins such as mycotoxins, further poisoning the tissues involved and spreading through the blood to affect other tissues.

Malnutrition

Acid accumulation impairs gut function through a number of mechanisms. Movement of the bowel is impaired, digestive enzyme production through the pancreas and the lining of the small bowel is reduced, and the more acid accumulates, the harder it is for the stomach lining to make enough new acid to digest food. The manufacturing of very strong acid requires a lot of energy, which is only possible when the body is functioning relatively well and is relatively alkaline overall. An acid body also has a much harder time detoxing because of impairment of the detox organs such as the liver and kidneys, resulting in excessive accumulation of toxins further impairing digestion and absorption. The organisms mentioned in the previous paragraph also rob the body of essential nutrients. The result is mal-

nutrition. In other words, trace minerals, vitamins, and antioxidants are usually grossly deficient in these circumstances (micronutrient malnutrition). Malnutrition caused by poor absorption—also acid related.

The majority of people have serious problems absorbing the nutrients that they take in because of an obstructive layer of mucus (biofilm) that forms in the gut starting from the stomach down to the large bowel. In the stomach, this layer of mucus is critical for protection of the stomach lining against the very acids and enzymes that are formed by the mucous membrane in order to digest food. Absence of this mucous layer leads to irritation and ultimately ulceration of the stomach wall. However, excessive mucus production resulting from poor diet, excessive acidity, increased toxin load in the food, insufficient enzymes for digestion, environmental pollution, lack of exercise, and even increased emotional stress can and does interfere with the ability of the gut to absorb nutrients and the ability of the gut to excrete waste and toxins efficiently. Biofilm is a glycoprotein (protein with sugar side-chains) produced by bacteria and certain other microbes in the body, especially those in the gut lining and adds to the mucous layer produced by the human mucin-producing cells lining the gut.

This mucous layer forms as a protective mechanism, especially under circumstances of excessive acidity and especially as a result of the intake of significant amounts of mucus-forming foods. The worst culprit foods include wheat, dairy, corn, all processed grains, alcohol, coffee, simple sugars, partially hydrogenated fats, and other animal proteins. Also, foods that have preservatives, artificial sweeteners, and other man-made chemicals in them encourage increased mucus production.

This mucous layer, which is thick, sticky, and cloudy literally forms a false lining in the gut that makes it hard for nutrients such as vitamins, minerals, and proteins (amino acids) to get absorbed efficiently. The benefit is that it binds toxins in order to facilitate their elimination from the body but in excess can cause a lot of problems. Biofilm produced by the microbes and human gut-produced mucin

also creates an ideal environment for the overgrowth of microorganisms such as fungus, yeast, bacteria, and parasites, which, in turn, produce more toxins that suppress the growth of good bacteria in the gut. These toxins get absorbed into the body affecting other areas directly and indirectly. They also eventually impact on transit time through the lower bowel leading to constipation, which is extremely common. Lack of fiber in the diet and a deficiency of good bacteria in the gut make this situation worse leading to more malnutrition. These "good bugs" that we need are responsible for making numerous critical nutrients such as folic acid, biotin, and vitamins B6, B12, B1, and K. All of this toxin load puts major stress on the lymphatic system, liver, and kidneys, which then have to deal with these toxins. The worst-case scenario is that these organisms can literally invade through the bowel and get into the bloodstream, leading to infections elsewhere in the body.

The microbial biofilm forms not only along the gut lining, but also in the blood vessels, causing dysfunction of the lining of the blood vessels, contributing to blood vessel malfunction. This malfunction contributes to the development of diseases such as hypertension and cholesterol plaque buildup, which, in turn, can lead to hardening of the arteries (atherosclerosis and coronary artery disease). It is now widely recognized that infectious organisms, mainly bacteria and viruses, contribute greatly to the development of conditions like atherosclerosis, which often lead to myocardial infarctions (heart attacks) and strokes. These organisms thrive inside and behind this biofilm.

In order to restore health, it is critical to get rid of the biofilm in the gut and inside blood vessels. We will discuss the solutions to this problem in a later section. We also will discuss key solutions to the acid-alkaline imbalances that contribute so much to the development of illness.

The Low-Fat Diet Health Myth

In the last couple of decades, we have been indoctrinated systematically with another myth, which is that fat in food is a major contributor to ill health. A multibillion-dollar food industry has been built around this myth, which up until very recently was supported by the US government and the medical community.

While it is true that certain fats can be unhealthy or even downright dangerous, i.e., partially hydrogenated fats; healthy fats form a critical part of a healthy diet and have very little to do with the obesity and chronic disease epidemic. Far more damaging is the idea that so-called "low-fat" foods that are high in processed complex carbohydrates and simple sugars or complex carbohydrates and artificial sweeteners are somehow healthier for us than more wholesome foods that contain healthy fats.

Inactivity

Inactivity is another aspect of lifestyle that is important and is contributing to the chronic disease epidemic. We have become a nation of physically inactive people with too many conveniences that make life too easy. We hardly have to leave the couch in front of our television. We can literally call in anything to us, including groceries. If you have a working right thumb and a working mouth, you can accomplish almost anything. Christopher Reeve was a prime example and did extraordinary things with great physical limitations. So is Stephen Hawking, one of the great astronomers of our time. He has been wheelchair-bound for more than twenty years because of an illness called ALS, but he knows more about black holes and quantum physics than any other human being alive. However, for the rest of us who are not quadriplegic in a wheelchair, if we don't use it, we lose it. It is a great travesty that even as we are less threatened by natural calamities and predators, we are more threatened by our dysfunctional lifestyles and habits.

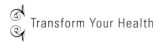

Sleep and Relaxation

Over 50 percent of Americans are sleep-deprived, with an estimated 60 million suffering from insomnia. Daytime sleepiness, difficulty concentrating, and impairment of memory are just some of the consequences of not getting enough sleep. Studies also have confirmed that sleep deprivation is a major contributor to the obesity epidemic that we are facing.

Stress and problems sleeping go hand in hand, leading to a large-scale increase in the levels of stress hormones in the body, including adrenaline and cortisone. The production of other hormones is suppressed when sleep deprivation occurs, including human growth hormone, a critical antiaging hormone, and DHEA (dihydroepiandrosterone), produced by the adrenal glands. Leptin levels also drop, which has an adverse effect on fat cell metabolism and appetite, increasing the likelihood of developing obesity. Melatonin production also suffers, which impairs the body's ability to repair itself. Melatonin is a key antioxidant hormone produced by the pineal gland and is also responsible for the normal body rhythms like the adrenal circadian rhythm. Low leptin levels also lead to permanent damage to a key part of the brain called the hippocampus. This, in turn, causes permanent memory impairment. Damage to the hippocampus is also a key component in the pathology leading to Alzheimer's disease.

Getting too little sleep also contributes to the suppression of our immune systems and reduces killer cell activity, which increases risk of cancer and increases our susceptibility to a number of infections. Leading contributors to sleep deprivation include the following:

1. A twenty-four-seven society: This is one of the consequences of modern society. Too much to do, and too little time. Nighttime, which used to be primarily focused on rest and recuperation, is now filled with entertainment or work that often lasts until the wee hours of the morning. The number of entertainment

Transform Your Life

choices is now almost unlimited, and many are available twenty-four hours a day.

2. Too much to do: Not only do we have unlimited entertainment options, but many of us are also deluged with work responsibilities at home as well as on the job. Many people work more than one job, and many often take work home. Most of us also spend tremendous amounts of time on tasks that are not urgent or important. Stephen Covey in his book, *First Things First* describes this issue well and how we can reprioritize in order to thrive.

3. Poor sleep habits: This goes with the issues described above, but in addition, many of us simply don't understand how much sleep we really need in order to function optimally. Sleep deficiency is becoming a problem even in our childhood population, especially among teens and young adults. We also don't seem to have an appreciation for how our brain works in terms of sleep. For example, watching television just before bedtime stimulates beta wave activity in the brain and tends to make it harder to fall asleep when we finally go to bed.

4. Obstacles in the bedroom: There are certain factors, such as light and sound pollution, electromagnetic field pollution, geopathic stress, allergens like dust mites in our pillows and mattresses, and television watching in bed, that can have very detrimental effects on our ability to get sufficient and good quality sleep.

5. Chemical interference: What we ingest before bedtime or even earlier affects our ability to sleep. Beverages and foods containing caffeine, sugar or artificial sweeteners can interfere with sleep up to twelve hours after being consumed. Many of us don't even know what or how much of these chemicals are in the products that we consume because we have not looked at the labels.

6. Hormonal culprits: Large numbers of our population live in adrenal overdrive because of stress and destructive habits, including those described above. The chronic fight-or-flight reactions cause the adrenal glands to pump out excessive amounts of adrenaline and other stress hormones and tend to suppress health-promoting hormones, like melatonin, which is produced by the pineal gland. All this creates a domino effect of adverse hormonal and health consequences.

7. "My head won't stop": Many of us are plagued by circling thoughts that don't want to stop when we go to bed. This is another consequence of stress and overstimulation. Anxiety and fear are two of the main culprits, with other negative emotions, such as guilt, sadness, and anger, also often coming into play.

8. Unresolved conflicts: Behind every health issue, including insomnia, is an underlying unresolved conflict that programs for the disease or symptom. Insomnia is synonymous with the conflict active phase when the sympathetic nervous system dominates. I will expand on this further in the second part of this book, "The Roots of Illness and Pathway to Wellness."

Getting too little sleep for extended periods of time for whatever reason is a major contributor to ill health in our society and needs to be addressed and resolved in order to heal.

Toxic Environment

A lot of us blame the environment for making us sick. It is true that we are breathing in and consuming through our food and water a larger number of toxins than ever before. There are close to 100,000 different man-made chemicals that are polluting our environment today, with thousands of new ones being added each year, and a large number of these are possibly harmful to the human body. Less than 10 percent of these chemicals have ever been studied to evaluate their effects on living organisms, and the vast majority of the studies that have been done are woefully inadequate in discerning the long-term consequences of exposure. There are, however, a substantial number of these chemicals that have been shown to be carcinogenic or damaging to the body in one way or another.

Fortunately, not all news regarding the environment is bad news. In some ways, our environment is actually doing better. For example, medium and large particulate air pollution has actually decreased. This is especially true in larger cities, where it is lower than it has been in over a hundred years because of pollution control measures that have been instituted over the past few decades. Also, the water supply is cleaner than it's ever been in our cities, but cleaner does not necessarily mean clean enough. In some ways, we have even backtracked by adding poisons such as fluoride and chlorine to our water supply.

The bottom line is that environmental pollution plays a vital role in what is making us sick, especially when accompanied by other factors such as poor diet, inadequate water intake, stress, and nega-

Transform Your Health

tive emotions in general. What is ironic is that environmental toxicity is often worse indoors than outdoors. It is well established that indoor pollution is becoming a bigger and bigger problem as energy efficiency has improved due to better insulation of our indoor environments at home, at work and even in the vehicles we drive. The sources of this pollution are numerous and include dry walls, carpets, electric wire insulation, paints, vinyl blinds and siding, furniture, and toxic house-cleaning products, just to mention a few.

Petroleum byproducts are another source of great concern. For example, one group of toxins commonly found in our food supply comes from plastics and is called phthalates (plasticizers). More and more of what we eat and drink these days comes in plastic, including the containers and the wrapping. Phthalates may be a major culprit, for example, in the obesity epidemic afflicting more and more people around the world and also may be a major contributor to a slew of other health problems, especially those associated with obesity.

Petroleum byproducts also are found in a variety of other products that we are commonly exposed to, including cosmetics, shampoos, soaps, lotions, lubricants, paint, pesticides, and even in the coating of some time-released medications. The US government just released a report acknowledging for the first time that toxins related to plastics are becoming a major contributor to health problems in this country. These toxins also are contributing to a blurring of the genders due to the adverse impacts substances like phthalates are having on hormone production in both men and women. These toxins often are described as being members of a group of toxins called xenoestrogens because of their hormone-like effects, which are very destructive. These chemicals are the main reason why more and more men are starting to look like women and women are starting to look more like men in body shape. We are becoming a nation of androgynous beings.

When you look at the waistlines of men and women, they are becoming rounder and rounder. These very toxins have estrogenic or hormonal-like effects that can cause weight gain in the central regions of the body leading to this shape shifting. In addition, we are

seeing a feminizing effect on the male population with characteristics such as impotence, breast enlargement, and shrinking genitalia. We are seeing women becoming more masculine with increased facial hair growth, deeper voices, and in both sexes, we are seeing a loss of libido. There has also been dramatic decrease in sperm counts in a large percentage of the male population and more problems with infertility in women. These effects are not solely caused by plastic toxicity but by other toxins as well that have hormone-like effects disrupting hormonal balances.

Other environmental toxins affecting our health include pesticides, herbicides, fungicides, heavy metals such as mercury, etc. Whole books have been written on the subject of environmental toxicity and the impact on health.

Water-based Toxicity

It is important to realize that a lot of toxicity comes into the human body through the water and other liquids that we consume. Even in a country like ours, where water standards are pretty high, it leaves a lot to be desired. A lot of pollutants are not filtered out of water properly because it's too hard or too expensive. This could only be done if we had reverse osmosis treatment plants on a mass scale, which would be prohibitively costly. It also would be somewhat counterproductive because of the elimination of salts and minerals from the water that the body needs.

Toxins that we commonly see in the water include heavy metals, pesticides, herbicides, medications, solvents, and other petrochemical pollutants. Water companies and water filtration plants in cities and towns around the country do a relatively good job in filtering out particulates and larger infectious organisms, such as most parasites, but they add chlorine in order to kill bacteria, smaller parasites and viruses. This chlorine when ingested is toxic in itself. Another toxic substance that is added to the water supply of most cities and towns in America is fluoride. There is little evidence of any significant ben-

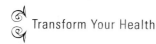

efit provided by fluoride but a large body of evidence showing that it has the potential to contribute significantly to ill health.

Water-based toxins also include chemicals like heavy metals, with lead and mercury being at the forefront. We do a relatively good job in the United States limiting the amounts of these toxins to relatively low doses, especially since lead was banned as a structural component of water pipes. Other materials that are used to make water pipes also can be toxic, including plastics and copper. Copper is normally not a problem, but there are small percentages of people that have a genetic disorder where they are unable to process copper and can get sick even from the copper released from water pipes.

We also are seeing pollution in our drinking water from pharmaceuticals used in treating humans and animals. These drugs are washed into the groundwater and into streams and lakes and then make it to our tap water because they cannot be filtered out. This includes medications such as Prozac (antidepressant), Premarin (female synthetic hormone), and acetaminophen; i.e., Tylenol. The amount of these medications in the drinking waters is extremely low (a fraction of what would normally be prescribed to patients), yet there is some evidence that even microscopic amounts of these can have an adverse effect on animal life.

More and more people are drinking bottled water because of the concerns they have with the city water supply. Unfortunately, most of them may not be doing themselves a favor. It has been shown that most bottled water is nothing more than city water with the chlorine filtered out, bottled in toxic plastic with an acid pH. The acidity alone can create huge health issues and should be addressed. Not only are we affected by the water we drink but even by the water we bathe, shower or swim in. Up to 70 percent of the toxins that come into our bodies from tap water come in through the skin and only 30 percent through the mouth.

Air Pollution

A lot of people think that air pollution is not a significant problem, whereas others think that it is a huge problem. I think that the truth lies somewhere in between. We have seen a marked improvement in the quality of air in the United States, especially in some of the largest cities, such as Los Angeles, Houston, and New York, where air pollution used to be extremely bad. It's still important to realize that we are exposed to literally thousands of different chemicals in the air that we breathe both indoors and outdoors. When people go indoors, they think they are safe from pollutants that may be floating around outside. Indoor air is typically five times more toxic than outside air. Indoor pollutants include particles and toxins released from wall paints, particleboard, new furniture, and so on. Add household chemicals to this, such as ammonium and aerosol sprays, furniture sprays, room deodorants, and insect sprays—all of which can be very hard on the body and very irritating to the upper airways and can contribute to various health conditions such as vasomotor rhinitis and asthma. It is much better to use natural household cleaning products rather than toxic ones.

Other pollutants that are worthy of a mention include radon gas, which pollutes homes across the country and often is far worse in the most energy-efficient homes. Energy efficiency is great for saving on electrical bills but also great in terms of trapping indoor pollutants and not allowing them to escape. Fortunately, there are methods available in which indoor air can be treated that will help to eliminate these toxins. These methods will be discussed in later chapters.

Another pollutant that can occur just about anywhere, especially indoors, is secondhand tobacco smoke. It is certainly a significant issue, especially when it comes to the very young and the very old, who are at much greater risk for or much more vulnerable to damage from this avoidable toxin.

This book is not meant to be an exhaustive reference on all possible toxins that people might come across. The object here is to

Transform Your Health

mention some of the most common so we can at least think in broad terms about what is happening to us and what is making us sick, and most importantly, what's at the root of health challenges and what can be done to resolve them.

Big Pharma

The pharmaceutical industry ("Big Pharma") is the second-most profitable industry on the face of the earth today (with a profit margin of 17.7 percent, compared with an average of only 2.5 percent for all industries), being beaten out only by the oil giants of the world (with a profit margin of 19.8 percent). This is a remarkable achievement by the pharmaceutical industry, which started from nothing about eighty years ago. When the history of the pharmaceutical industry is reviewed, it becomes readily apparent how its power has grown by leaps and bounds over these eighty years. It is now at the point where it dominates the health care industry, not only because physicians cannot practice without its support, but also because of its influence on the multiple layers of bureaucracies that make decisions on the direction that health care is taking.

The pharmaceutical industry in the United States employs more political lobbyists and spends more than $855 million per year on lobbying. Both are more than any other industry. It also employs over one hundred thousand pharmaceutical representatives pursuing 120,000 prescribers. This means that for every one prescriber, there is close to one drug representative. Each representative's full-time job is to convince that prescriber to write prescriptions for its company's drugs. Each year 3.4 billion prescriptions are written, bringing in a profit that now averages over $275 billion per year. These profits have increased 250 percent over the past decade because drug prices have more than doubled and because more people are taking the drugs. The top ten companies worldwide account for over 44

Transform Your Health

percent of that profit. Eight of these top ten companies are for-eign-owned; however, half of their drug profits are made from US consumers.

This industry started taking off in the 1920s and '30s, when pen-icillin and insulin first hit the market. It was a minor player until the 1950s, when the rules governing the drug industry were rewritten to give individual companies wide protections against competition. In the 1970s, drug prices really started taking off after legislation was passed, giving the pharmaceutical industry even bigger advantages and greater influence over the prescribing habits of health care pro-fessionals. The industry has consistently claimed the need for these extraordinary rules to ensure greater profitability in order to do the research and development on new drugs. The irony is that phar-maceutical companies actually spend less money on research and development than other industries that are far less profitable. On the other hand, the pharmaceutical industry spends far more on sales and marketing and lobbying than any other industry.

"Me Too" Drugs

The drug industry claims that it is spending billions of dollars attemping to develop new drugs that are going to save mankind, and yet only a tiny fraction of the drugs that have been released into the marketplace are new at all. The vast majority of so-called new drugs are "me too" drugs that are basically minor variations on drugs already on the market. In most cases, these are no more effective than the old drugs they compete against.

Influence on Science

Is it possible that drug companies actually skew the results from research on the drugs that they make to show greater effects and benefits than are real? A recent meta-analysis of studies sponsored by drug companies shows that drug company-sponsored drug stud-

ies are several times more likely to show positive results than studies sponsored by organizations not affiliated with those drug companies. As a scientist, if the hand that feeds you is the same one sponsoring your research, you may have an inclination to do what you could to show the best face possible on such sponsor's drugs. Pharmaceutical companies are under no obligation to publish studies that show that their drugs don't work. All they have to do is avoid publicity of negative results while publicizing those that are positive.

Reasons to Be Concerned

1. Drugs treat symptoms, not diseases. They often facilitate disease progression and contribute to the development of new diseases.

2. Health care costs are bankrupting our society. The rise in medical costs is unsustainable, and the biggest contributor to these rapidly rising costs is rising drug prices and over-prescribing.

3. Innovation is being stifled because of the huge influence of the drug industry on the health care field. Only a fraction of the money spent on research goes for non-drug therapies compared to drug therapies.

4. Proven, natural therapies and those who administer them are being suppressed by the drug industry because of its extraordinary influence on the medical industry, insurance industry, the media, and our politicians.

5. Media influence of the drug industry makes it nearly impossible for the voices of those promoting non-drug therapies, such as those found in natural medicine, to be heard. The public is left with the impression that drugs are the only game in town.

6. Politicians are heavily influenced by this industry. The pharmaceutical industry is very closely tied to

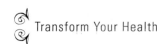

the political structures in this country. This industry contributes extremely large amounts of money to the election campaigns of politicians on both sides of the political divide in the United States. It is playing both sides to ensure that no one will attempt to mess with its power structure and its control of health care.

7. The pharmaceutical industry also has great influence on the medical organizations that run medicine in this country through the industry's sponsorship of everything from the organizations themselves to educational seminars that are given to physicians and medical students. The industry also makes large financial contributions to medical schools and medical libraries. It has its financial finger in every pot. It, therefore, becomes very difficult for any of these organizations to stand up to the pharmaceutical industry when it oversteps its bounds.

8. Insurance companies are also tied into this sinister network and are heavily influenced by the drug companies. They are generally strongly discouraged from creating insurance policies that would support patient choice, especially when patient choice involves alternative medicine, integrative medicine, or anything that falls outside of the conventional box. By refusing to pay for anything but conventional diagnostic workups and treatments, they basically control consumer health care choices. The vast majority of consumers feel they have no choice but to get care from a conventional health care system focused on treating symptoms with toxic drugs rather than finding and treating their causes.

Big Pharma to the Rescue

Again, I do not want to leave the impression that Big Pharma is all bad and evil. There is a strong case to be made for the good that this industry has done for society. In certain areas, Big Pharma has made a huge difference by developing dozens of life-saving drugs that have made a tremendous difference in the management of acute, life-threatening illnesses. With the discovery of penicillin, for example, a revolution was set in motion that brought about a fundamental shift in health care. All of a sudden, in our society, people did not have to worry constantly about infections cutting their life short or taking their children from them before their time. When penicillin was discovered, it instantly changed the face of a large number of infectious diseases that were untreatable at the time, except for supportive care, which relied on the patient's immune system to fight off the infection successfully.

Another great advance in medicine was the discovery of insulin and the ability to extract it and inject it into humans. This gave diabetics a new lease on life and meant that they could live full, relatively healthy lives, whereas shortly before, they were doomed to die within a year or two after the diagnosis was made, depending on the severity of the disease.

Double-edged Sword

Big Pharma also revolutionized the treatment of conditions like pain and inflammation and with the advent of steroids almost overnight gave relief to large numbers of people who were struggling with severe aches and pains in joints, muscles, and tendons. Unfortunately, it took a good ten to fifteen years before there was a full realization as to the downside of these wonder drugs. It was discovered that people were dying by the thousands from preventable chronic illnesses because of steroid side effects. These side effects included rampant osteoporosis, development of diabetes, immune system dysfunction, and escalating weight gain. These drugs also

led to the collapse of adrenal function in patient after patient as their own production of adrenal hormones shut down in the face of overwhelming doses of steroids. This led to a very dramatic change in medicine, with the focus changing to drugs that had less severe side effects but were still very effective in the treatment of inflammation. This group was called nonsteroidal anti-inflammatory drugs (NSAIDs), and with the advent of these drugs, like aspirin, ibuprofen, and others that are now freely available over the counter, made another tremendous difference in the treatment of musculoskeletal diseases (diseases of the skeleton and muscles).

However, again, it took many disasters, including the deaths of thousands of people, to awaken us to the fact that these drugs were doing some really nasty things, including creating bleeding stomach erosions and kidney damage. Some of these drugs were taken off the market many years ago because of the destruction they were causing. Rofecoxib (Vioxx) is one in particular. The FDA estimates that Vioxx was implicated in the deaths of at least 28,000 people in the United States. The Financial Times reported in January 2005 that FDA experts had publicly acknowledged a much higher death toll linked to this drug. Their estimates reportedly place the death toll at between 89,000 and 140,000 in the United States and as many as 200,000 worldwide. It took six years from the time it was released into the market before it was withdrawn. In spite of the high complication rate and the high death toll, the FDA reapproved Vioxx in 2005. Because of the legal ramifications, the manufacturer (Merck) has kept it off the market. Vioxx was one of the nonsteroidal anti-inflammatory drugs to come along that was supposed to be safe because it caused fewer stomach problems. But little did we know that it would cause other problems, such as an increased incidence of myocardial infarctions (heart attacks), congestive heart failure, or stroke.

This drug may come back on the market, even though it may be responsible for a large number of deaths, because consumers are being led to believe that there are no alternatives. Insurance companies won't pay for many alternatives, so consumers allegedly pres-

sured the FDA into reapproving this drug in spite of its deadly legacy. The only difference is it will carry black box warnings regarding the risk of deadly side effects. The warnings will relieve the company of future liability when more people die.

Most people don't know that many great alternatives to these deadly drugs exist. These alternatives are often as effective or more effective and have none of the very deadly side effects. In the rare incidence of side effects, they tend to be mild. Again, when you treat the root of the problem and support recovery through natural means, the outcome is usually far more satisfactory.

Selling Sickness

When you look at people who are the healthiest in our society and who live the longest, there are numerous things that they have in common. One major factor seems to be that they are far less likely to take medications of any kind on a regular basis. Some may argue that they take fewer drugs because they are healthier in the first place. However, it also can be argued that they live longer because they are exposed to far fewer symptom-focused drugs that contribute to disease formation by impairing the body's natural defense mechanisms. Taking pharmaceuticals can be characterized as a slippery slope where taking one drug leads to side effects requiring a second drug, leading to more side effects and ever more drugs at higher doses. In this manner, we become more and more impaired health wise, falling victim to more and more disease labels.

The list of diseases also is constantly expanding, with people previously deemed healthy now being classified as ill with one or more of these newly named diseases. What were previously judged to be normal symptoms pointing to the internal adjustments a body makes to constant change within and outside of our bodies are now being tagged with new disease labels.

A Slippery Slope

Let's step back and look at this in more detail. On average, when somebody goes to a physician today for a routine checkup, he is doing his due diligence and getting "preventive care." He gets his

exam and often gets a clean bill of health. Blood pressure is "normal." Lungs and heart and every other organ system that can be felt or listened to are normal as the physician does his cursory superficial examination, which takes in most cases less than a minute. Blood sugar is "normal." Blood chemistries are "normal." By the way, "normal" means that your values fall in the range where 90 percent of the population is, which unfortunately is a far cry from what could be called optimal blood levels, i.e., compared with those in ideal health. I would say "normal" is overrated if you realize where most "normal" people are as far as their health is concerned. Do you really want to be where 90 percent of the population currently is health wise?

So you return a year later for your routine annual examination. This time the physician turns around and tells you that even though you were perfectly "normal" last year, this year you have a disease that needs to be treated. Then he gives it a name, and the name might be real simple, like high blood pressure, or hypertension, or maybe even diabetes. And, of course, most of the time they slap you with this new label, without batting an eye, that you will carry thenceforth for the rest of your life. You now take on the mass consciousness that is represented by this label—the history of that illness, how it tends to respond to treatment, how people feel when they have this disease, what people do in terms of drugs and other medical treatments when they have this disease, and how many people die from this disease. All of that in one fell swoop lands right on your head without you even realizing it. You are now given a prescription that you are told will need to be taken for this particular illness for the rest of your life. Often when you first get the prescription, you don't even realize it will be a lifelong commitment because the communication between you and the physician is often minimal. The physician only has about five or ten minutes to tell you about this curse that you are now saddled with for the rest of your life. And in passing, he might mention that you may think about changing your lifestyle, eating habits, and include some exercise, as if this mantra is going to somehow inspire you to make radical changes to your lifestyle.

They give you the prescription with a list of adverse effects that might be anticipated. When you look at the full list, fear takes hold or at least some concern because there is a whole gamut of side effects, including possible death. How do you feel about taking something that might kill you? Of course, you are between a rock and a hard place because on the one hand, the disease can kill you. On the other hand, the drug might also do you in. So what do you do? You go right ahead into the abyss with an enemy on each side—walking to the gallows.

Sure enough, most people have some side effects. Often they don't even realize that they are having side effects, because the side effects don't start immediately in most cases. Sometimes the side effects don't even start the day after, two days after, or even a week after. Usually, they happen gradually over time. For example, a very common side effect of the vast number of pharmaceutical drugs on the market for everything from hypertension to diabetes is weight gain.

So do most people connect the weight gain of twenty pounds with a drug that they started three months ago? Unfortunately, out of ignorance, most people don't make the connection. They go to the physician, and they complain about the weight gain, and they are told, "Sorry, sir (or ma'am), you are getting older, and your metabolism is slowing down" or "you are just eating too much and getting too little exercise. That's just one of those things that you will have to deal with." So you continue taking your drug and experience more and more side effects. The sad thing is that your new problem of obesity links to other problems, including the worsening of the health problem that you were struggling with in the first place, such as hypertension.

You soon find that you cannot control this particular symptom with one drug, so the physician starts the merry-go-round with more drugs. He changes you to one drug or another, and keeps adding as he goes. The easiest path is just to add because attempting to figure out what's the best drug will be just as frustrating for the physician and patient alike. So as the patient continues going through this gauntlet the side effects continue to mount without the patient

ever realizing it—because, again, they didn't start the day the patient started the drugs. They started over time and progressed slowly. In an amazing way, we are literally creating disease in our society left and right. Not only that, but pharmaceutical companies, in conjunction with their company-sponsored medical organizations and medical schools, are constantly expanding the list of diseases with a list of old and new drugs to treat these diseases. Then they spend millions of dollars educating the public through direct advertising to the public and by sponsoring support groups and organizations for lay people to "educate" the public on these new diseases and the drugs recommended for them.

Selling People on New Diseases

The way that a new disease is created is by getting people and their physicians to buy into the idea that something that used to be seen as a normal part of life or a normal internal response to a constantly changing internal or external environment—like, for example, PMS or mild to moderate anxiety or depression—should be classified as a disease with an imposing new label. For example, symptoms such as moodiness or tearfulness combined with water retention and headaches is now called premenstrual dysphoric disorder (PMDD) instead of PMS, and instead of recommending common sense approaches, such as dietary adjustments and reducing stress, physicians now recommend antidepressants, birth control pills, and/or diuretics. This simple reclassification has opened up another potential multi-billion dollar profit center for these pharmaceutical companies, especially seeing that a large percentage of women around the world are now candidates for drug treatment under this new classification.

A long list of new diseases has been created over the past fifteen to twenty years in a similar manner. I'm not implying that there is no basis for these new so-called disease entities. But what I am saying is that when a drug company needs to create new profit centers by expanding the use of its existing drugs or by developing new drugs, the easiest way to do it is to pair these drugs with new diseases.

On the other hand, there is far more competition already in place if they focus on developing new treatments for diseases that have been around for a long time, with many other drugs already available for the treatment of that disease. A good example would be a disease like hypertension.

Selling Symptoms as Diseases

The conventional medical profession and the drug companies that they are entangled with love to take symptoms, such as high blood pressure, high cholesterol, or high blood sugar, and turn them into diseases. Once these symptoms are labeled as diseases, the drug companies have open season on creating drugs to treat them without ever really having to pay attention to the underlying factors causing the symptom. For example, over thirty years ago, a correlation was found between coronary artery disease and high cholesterol. The medical community and drug companies immediately jumped to the conclusion that high cholesterol must be the cause of coronary artery disease and started creating drugs to treat high cholesterol. As a result, the cholesterol drug market is now the most lucrative and profitable of all drug categories.

Come to find out, high cholesterol is not the enemy that we used to think it was. As a matter of fact, cholesterol is a critical nutrient that plays a critical role in the function of every cell in the body, both as a key ingredient of the cell membrane and as a critical precursor to all the sex hormones and most of the adrenal hormones in the body. Cholesterol levels do go up when the body is stressed or overloaded with toxins because the liver makes more of it in order to protect the cells in the liver, increase the production of stress hormones, and in order to patch injured blood vessels. It is actually inflammation and oxidation in the blood vessels and the activation of clotting mechanisms that normally lead to heart attacks, not high cholesterol alone. As a matter of fact, it is well known that more than half of the people who die of heart attacks had normal or low cholesterol levels when they had their fatal heart attack. It turns out that a

Transform Your Life

certain group of drugs called statin drugs, used in the treatment of high cholesterol, do lower the risk of a second heart attack, mainly because they actually mitigate the inflammation of the inner lining of the blood vessels. Other drugs that only treat high cholesterol and not inflammation have never been shown to lower the risk of heart attacks. As a matter of fact, some of them are even correlated with a slight increase in risk when taking these drugs.

The problem with the statin drugs is they have other side effects, such as the weakening of muscles, including the heart muscle, which is correlated with a dramatic rise in the incidence of congestive heart failure over the past twenty-five years. These drugs also are implicated in the increased incidence of depression, accidents, impotence (lowers testosterone levels in men), forgetfulness, fatigue, and even cancer (low cholesterol levels are correlated with an increased risk of cancer).

For example, the statin drugs are known to deplete the body of a key nutrient that is essential for producing energy in every cell. This nutrient is called Coenzyme Q10. When Coenzyme Q10 levels are depleted, congestive heart failure ensues. The heart muscle gets weaker and weaker until it finally fails. As the incidence of myocardial infarctions has stabilized and even decreased slightly the incidence of congestive heart failure has dramatically increased since statin drugs were first introduced into the market in 1987. Within five years of the introduction of statin drugs the incidence of congestive heart failure started rising. This rise is continuing as more people are taking these drugs. I'm not saying that it is solely due to the statin drugs, but it is my contention and that of many other experts that statin drugs have a lot to do with it.

This is not all. When cholesterol is treated aggressively and cholesterol levels drop very low, it also contributes to a marked decrease in the production of certain hormones that the body manufactures from cholesterol including all sex hormones produced by the ovaries and the testicles and the adrenal hormones. Women, for example, frequently experience a decrease in their estrogen, progesterone, and testosterone levels; men tend to experience a decrease in their levels

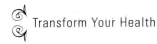

of testosterone and progesterone, and both men and women experience a decrease in their adrenal hormone levels including DHEA as well as a decrease in the levels of a critical hormone which is the precursor to all the sex and adrenal hormones listed above, called pregnenolone. This in turn contributes to a decrease in energy and sex drive and an increase in the incidence of erectile dysfunction, osteoporosis, chronic fatigue, depression, and memory problems. Some studies have even shown an increased risk of accidents and premature death from causes other than coronary artery disease. I'm not stating that these drugs cause these problems. I know that many factors go into the development of any illness, but it's certainly something we need to be concerned about and something we should be studying.

Other disease labels that have been added to the medical lexicon more recently that has led to a booming drug market to treat individuals diagnosed with it includes attention deficit hyperactivity disorder (ADHD). This diagnostic label was added in the 1980s and since then has led to multibillion-dollar annual drug sales to treat it with millions of children being treated for this condition. Millions of children in this country have been sentenced to a childhood and sometimes a lifetime of having to take stimulants ("speed"-like drugs) in order to treat this condition. Unfortunately once on them it is often very difficult to get these kids off these drugs and more and more of them are taking them into adulthood. The price our kids and adults pay for attempting to come off these drugs include severe fatigue that is very hard to treat. Many experts even in the conventional medical field feel that this diagnosis is way over used and that our kids are being thrown onto these drugs way to easily when behavioral modification strategies are often just as effective as drug treatment with none of the side effects. It is ironic that it is illegal to buy or sell amphetamines ("speed") in this country, and yet we have no problem putting millions of our kids and adults on speed-like stimulants.

Physicians Selling Sickness

Members of the medical profession that are licensed to prescribe drugs tend to be very quick on the trigger when it comes to labeling patients who are having symptoms with diagnoses which, in turn, helps justify the prescribing of pharmaceuticals to treat these symptoms. This represents by far the most efficient path to keep doctor visits as short as possible so that more patients can be squeezed in to their schedules. The average physician only spends nine minutes from beginning to end with each patient they see which is no where near enough time to really be able to figure out what is at the source of their patient's misery and what steps might be taken other than drug interventions to treat their symptoms.

Physicians are trained in medical school to be very efficient at reviewing the signs and symptoms that patients present to them so that a diagnosis can be made and the label can be given to the patient. The patient is then sold on this new label and the need for often expensive, side effect producing drugs that will need to be prescribed and taken for this newly diagnosed disease. Patients are often intimidated into doing what the physician tells them to do and to take what has been prescribed. The patient is warned that if the prescription is not filled and taken as prescribed that serious consequences may result—including death.

Pharmaceutical companies have become so brazen in their sales pitches that they now advertise directly to consumers. They have been able to convince millions of consumers to label themselves with diseases and for the consumers to then turn around and sell their physicians on what they are convinced is wrong with them and what drugs they would like to be treated with. They often get more than enough information from the media to make a pretty convincing case to their physicians that they need to be given a prescription for the advertised drug or drugs. (The United States is the only country that allows direct marketing of prescription drugs to the consumer.)

Why we should be careful about buying when others are selling sickness:

1. Being labeled with a disease may be dangerous to your health. A label can convince you that you are sicker than you really are and may even quicken your demise. This is especially true when you are diagnosed with a serious life-threatening illness and then labeled not just with the disease label but also with a prognosis that may not be favorable.

2. The drugs that are prescribed for all these new (and old) diseases can have serious side effects. As a matter of fact, it is worth being reminded that almost all drugs are foreign chemicals to the human body and tend to have side effects both short-term and long-term. There are so many examples that could be mentioned here, but I will limit it to just a handful to make my point.

   Certain drugs used in the treatment of conditions like diabetes, hypertension, and depression often make the disease that is being treated worse over time because of all the negative effects on metabolism. For example, the vast majority of diabetic medications and antidepressants, and quite a few drugs in the antihypertensive category, cause a slow down in metabolism, an increase in appetite, and a tendency toward significant weight gain. Again, this contributes to the development of a whole series of other conditions linked to obesity.

3. It can be very costly from a financial perspective. Direct out of pocket health care expenses and the cost of health insurance is considerable in this country. Prescription drug prices have been rising much more rapidly than inflation for decades and so has all forms of conventional medical care. Treating symptoms can be very expensive.

4. You may be ceding control of your health care choices to other so-called experts in the health care field that may not even have a clue what consequences their labels

and prescribed treatments may have on you and your health. By accepting the labels that these professionals dole out so freely you also tend to accept their treatments that often include very negative consequences.

Noncompliance

So, have you ever been labeled a noncompliant patient because you would not take the drug or drugs that you were prescribed? Maybe you wouldn't take them at all, or you wouldn't take them at the frequency recommended, or you wouldn't just keep on taking them even though you had some side effects or concerns about things, like weight gain, decreased energy, stomach disturbances, and so on.

If you are one of these people, you might just be saving your own life. I'm not promoting noncompliance here, but when you are treating the symptom and not the cause, you do so at your own peril. However, sometimes symptoms do need to be treated in conjunction with the cause, especially if the symptom is immediately life threatening. If your blood pressure is out of control, with your readings through the roof, it is true that you might run the risk of a sudden stroke or your heart giving out, risking possible catastrophe. However, if you were to pursue your drug regimens with zest and great compliance without getting to the source, chances are that you might end up with other illnesses.

Let us study a few examples of noncompliant behavior. Now, you will notice some people are noncompliant because they just don't care a hoot to follow anybody's instructions. They are pretty rebellious in spirit, and they just don't care about their health as much as their physician who is taking care of them does. And frankly, they may even be into a little bit of self-sabotage. Some are even tired of being on this planet and are ready to take the slow coach out (slow suicide).

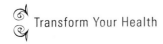

A second category of noncompliance is people that are noncompliant for good reasons, i.e., they may be punch-drunk on the fact that every time they take a drug, they have a side effect that puts them down for a few days or just makes them miserable. It might be an antidepressant that causes weight gain of thirty or forty pounds, yet the physician expects the patient to continue taking the drug regardless.

There is a third category of noncompliance, which consists of the people who are well-educated that have a deeper understanding of pathology or understand intuitively the fact that the illness was not caused by a drug deficiency, i.e., depression isn't caused by a Prozac deficiency. They feel there is another cause or another factor that is not being addressed, and they would rather experience the symptom to remind them that something is out of balance than just suppress it and override it summarily.

The fourth category of noncompliance is the people that disagree that they have an illness. Some of them disagree out of ignorance, and some have a deeper insight into the fact that they simply don't want to be labeled with diseases. Instead, they want to see where the symptoms point. Most of these people are operating out of intuition, because they don't have the knowledge and information presented, for example, in this book. But they have a feeling that it isn't their genes, and it isn't bad luck. There's something else at the source of their illness.

In summary, being a bit of a skeptic when it comes to being labeled with a disease, especially incurable ones, and when it comes to prescriptions for potentially dangerous and sometimes even potentially lethal drugs may save you from unnecessary misery and may even save your life. Blindly accepting disease labels without realizing the consequences of doing so and following the advice of those in the health care field that are trigger happy when it comes to throwing prescriptions at you without giving thought to the possible side effects may not always be such a good idea. The bottom line is, be careful what you buy into from those that are selling sickness.

Food Supply in Jeopardy

The foods we consume today are a far cry from those our forbearers consumed a hundred years ago. All categories of foods have changed tremendously through genetic engineering and processing. We certainly do not get the nutrient value from foods that were available when they were grown more naturally. There are now far more concerns about the safety and healthfulness of our food supply than ever before.

There are some things about our food supply, though, to be thankful for. Even though we still see some foodborne illnesses, they are few and far between, compared with the more distant past. For example, at the turn of the nineteenth century, it was extremely common to develop gastrointestinal conditions, such as gastroenteritis, related to food and waterborne infectious organisms. Today, that has changed dramatically, and very few people get gastrointestinal infections or food poisoning, and when they do, it is usually big news and leads to rapid government action to track down and withdraw contaminated products from the market.

GMO Foods

GMO is the abbreviation for genetically modified organisms. Genetic engineering was touted as a miracle when man first started manipulating the genetic code of certain plants that we eat. There are many good reasons why agricultural companies have encouraged this approach. Growing food in a cost-effective way, on a mass scale,

 Transform Your Health

is not an easy thing to accomplish. Genetic engineering has made it possible to manipulate plant growth in many different ways. Everything from the amount of water that plants need to be able to grow, to where they can be grown successfully, to increased resistance against common pests that can destroy those crops, to the speed at which they grow, to the size to which they grow, to even the flavor of the produce can be and have been manipulated. All of these are reasons why agricultural companies practice genetic engineering.

A very significant number of our most commonly consumed foods fall into the category of GMO foods now. Many of them are nearly impossible to find on our store shelves in non-GMO form these days. These include corn and soy, and the produce containing or made from these foods. There are numerous other common fruits and vegetables and even grains that are now, to a greater or lesser extent, in this category. Certain plants that have been genetically engineered (like wheat) grow fungi on them when they are stored. These fungi produce toxins called mycotoxins, which are very toxic to the human nervous system. One common wheat-borne mycotoxin has even been shown to have an LSD-like effect and can literally make you high. It also can cause withdrawal symptoms when wheat-based foods are eliminated from the diet. These are signs of serious addiction like you would expect to see with street drugs, but not with foods.

There are some other very serious consequences needing our urgent attention, including the fact that foods that are genetically engineered tend to be up to four or five times more allergenic than foods that are not genetically engineered. This is the case with corn, soy, and other plants. It is estimated that as many as 80 percent of people in America are sensitive to corn when tested through bioenergetic forms of testing, compared with only 20 percent in Mexico, where they still use non-GMO corn to a large extent. This is now changing rapidly because Mexico is importing a lot of its corn from America. Food sensitivities are discussed later in greater detail, but suffice it to say that they can translate to a lot of symptoms and exacerbation and even creation of illness.

Chemicals on Our Food

Almost all of the vegetables, fruits and grains commercially grown in this country are treated, sometimes multiple times before harvesting, with large amounts of pesticides and fungicides, which also contribute greatly to the poison load carried in our bodies and adversely affect our health. This is one reason for the growing popularity of the organic movement around the United States and many parts of the industrialized world. More and more people are realizing that they are being poisoned on a daily basis by what is being sprayed on their food and added to the soil.

This also applies to heavy metals, such as lead, mercury, arsenic, and even radioactive uranium that contaminates not only our water, but also food sources. Mercury-contaminated smog, originating from China's and India's thousands of coal-burning power stations, follows the prevailing winds to the United States and Canada and contaminates rainwater falling to earth. Uranium contamination also is becoming an ever-bigger problem because of all the nuclear activity around the globe, including nuclear weapons tests in countries such as India, Pakistan, and North Korea. High mercury levels, lead levels, and cadmium levels are also quite common.

Nutrient Deficiency and Depletion

Most people don't realize that when they make their best effort to change their lifestyle by eating more vegetables and fruits, for example, they are eating foods that are nutrient and energy deficient. The reason is that most land that is farmed today has been farmed on for a century or more. The soil has become depleted of essential minerals, such as iodine, chromium, selenium, manganese, magnesium, calcium, iron and more. When farmers fail to rotate crops properly, which helps to refresh and renew the soil, or when they fail to nurture the soil properly by adding more wholesome fertilizers, like compost or manure, containing key trace minerals, crops suffer, and our produce becomes more nutrient-deficient.

 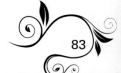

Our world has become such an interconnected place that our food sources come from across the globe and not just from up the road. It is now possible for companies to ship produce from the other side of the globe and still get it to you fresh enough to be consumable. However, fresh is a relative concept because fresh sometimes means that from the time that the produce is harvested until it is actually consumed can be as long as two to four weeks. Most fruits, for example, are picked green, boxed up, packaged, and shipped from the country of origin to other countries, some half a world away. Then they have to be unloaded, transferred to trucks, and transported to warehouses, where the produce is often gassed with methane to accelerate ripening. It is then delivered to grocery stores to be placed out on display, where it finally reaches the consumer, who depends on his produce lasting up to a few more days before he consumes it. A large percentage of produce these days is also treated with gamma ray radiation to destroy organisms that would normally accelerate spoilage.

The result of all this time delay from harvesting to consumption, and the fact that produce is often picked before it naturally ripens, leads to further nutrient depletion of the produce and a markedly diminished vitality rating. Vitality rating relates to the vital energy content (life force) inherent to all living organisms. For example, freshly picked fruits and vegetables have a very high vitality rating, whereas a hamburger with a bun made of devitalized, processed wheat, with a microwaved patty made from devitalized meat and soy, has a very low vitality rating. Any food that can be stored for a long time, especially at room temperature, is also likely to have a very low vitality rating. The higher the vitality rating of a vegetable or fruit, the quicker it will tend to spoil, but the better it is for your body.

Food Processing

Food that reaches the supermarket shelf and is not in its natural form is very likely to be bad for your health. Any food that is heavily processed with man-made chemicals added to help preserve it

or to help make it more flavorful or to improve its texture, and so on, is going to have a negative impact on your efforts to stay or get healthy.

The weight loss industry is just one example of an industry misleading the public on a massive scale in order to rake in huge profits on so-called diet foods and beverages. It is ironic that, over the last twenty years, we have gone through one diet craze after another, each being touted as the ultimate "cure" for obesity and always ending up in failure over the long-term. You may be able to cut calories by consuming these diet products, but because these products add to the toxin and acidity load in the body, they also slow metabolism to a crawl, thereby assuring that initial weight loss achieved, if any, will reverse itself usually sooner than later.

It is estimated that 95 percent of people with obesity will fail to maintain their weight loss, if they lost weight, over two years, and 98 percent of people will fail to maintain their weight loss over five years. One of the reasons for this shocking statistic is food processing. Other reasons have been presented in previous chapters. One key to being successful with any weight loss plan or health-recapturing program is to focus on eating healthy and avoiding processed and packaged foods unless there is ample evidence of their benefit. This means eating plenty of non-GMO foods with high vitality ratings and low levels of man-made toxins on or in them.

Are Your Vitamin Supplements Helping You?

Even the supplement industry is mistaken or even disingenuous when it claims that taking vitamins can replace healthy, energy-rich foods. Even the best vitamins on the market are low in terms of vitality rating. At best, they can assist you at increasing nutrient levels in a body that is severely depleted of certain nutrients in conjunction with a very healthy diet.

Vitamins extracted from unhealthy foods—i.e., most vitamin C on the market, which is extracted from GMO corn—can make things even worse by triggering food sensitivities to the supplement itself. In addition, a lot of supplements come with a dose of man-made toxin contained in the supplement itself because of the way that they are manufactured. For example, it is not unusual to find small amounts of solvent contamination in supplements. The reason for this is that companies that make supplements use machinery that has to be cleaned in between batches. Most of the companies don't have enough machinery to do every type of supplement on a different machine. So what do they do? They clean the machines in between batches with solvents that are not completely removed before the next batch is made. This, then, inadvertently gets into the batch of supplements made with that machine.

It is worth emphasizing the point that we better figure out what it is that we are consuming or else we will be putting ourselves at the mercy of unscrupulous peddlers of poison, trying to make a profit at any cost. The bottom line is, if you want to get healthy or stay healthy, stay away from processed food, eat organic as much as possible, or if you can't afford it, consider growing your own. Also be very careful of which supplements you choose to take. You may be doing yourself more harm than good!

Is Modern Technology Making Us Sick?

We live in an extraordinary era in the history of mankind. When you look around you, you stand in wonder of the tremendous advances that have been made in a very short period of time. The world is changing so fast technologically; it can make your head spin. These advances in technology are accompanied by extraordinary advances in our knowledge of our world, so much so that it is estimated that the overall global knowledge base literally doubles about every two years. Just imagine if you go to college to study medicine. By the time you finish the four years of medical school, more than half of what you have learned is probably outdated, especially in certain subjects.

With all of these advances in technology come some serious downsides that we urgently need to become familiar with before it is too late. We have already talked about chemical pollution of our air, water, and food supply, but there is another form of pollution that poses potentially serious threats to our health that very few of us are aware of. In fact, another conspiracy of silence reigns because of the economic interests involved.

Electrosmog, or electromagnetic field pollution, is one such serious threat to be aware of even though it is by no means the only aspect of modern technology that is hurting us health wise. Electrosmog, which now affects every corner of the globe is especially problematic in industrialized countries and is worse in highly popu-

lated areas. We are bombarded by waves of electromagnetic energy that our bodies were never meant to experience. Cell towers are popping up on every other corner, satellites are circling the globe in the hundreds, and radar stations monitoring the weather and airplanes are bombarding us with electromagnetic waves. Microwave ovens blast food that we put into our bodies, radiating our intestinal tracts indirectly. When we stand close to these devices while they are operating, we get radiated directly as well. Cell phones radiate our brains while we are conversing with others, and the rest of the body is radiated just by carrying the phones on or near our bodies. Even the electrical wiring in our homes and overhead power lines and transformers close to our homes and businesses are affecting us.

More and more studies are coming out (many of them unpublished) showing how we are being negatively affected. The telecommunications industry is bigger and more powerful than the pharmaceutical and food industries combined and certainly has a vested interest in keeping us in the dark as far as the detrimental health effects of telecommunications systems.

Fritz-Albert Popp, the leading expert internationally on quantum physics and more specifically on biophotonics, has demonstrated unequivocally with his one-of-a-kind bio-photon camera the effects of certain ranges of electromagnetic radiation on living organisms. The body is surrounded by a bio-photon sphere that interacts with the body and is responsible for communication between cells along a network of structures called tubulin, where information to and in between cells travels at the speed of light. This "light body" and the DNA of the cells interact and communicate. DNA vibrates at several billion hertz per second. In other words, the DNA molecular coil extends and contracts at this rate and releases one single photon each time it contracts. (A photon is a unit of light.) These photons communicate with bio-photons in a highly structured light field around the body. This, in turn, regulates activity of metabolic enzymes responsible for all biochemical activity in the cells. The receiver in the cell is the structure called tubulin, which conducts the

Transform Your Life

bio-photons. By the way, the heavy metal mercury destroys tubulin and, thereby, disrupts communication between cells.

It seems that electromagnetic radiation that corresponds in frequency to the frequency by which DNA vibrates is the most harmful. Number one on that list is cordless phones and then, in descending order, wireless Internet, cell phones when used against the ear, bluetooth technologies, EMF in the house from TVs, computer monitors, laptop computers, alarm clocks, electrical wiring in the walls and ceilings, cell towers, radar stations, and satellite transmissions.

Dr. Dietrich Klinghardt, who is one of the leading figures in alternative and integrative medicine, has demonstrated the effects of electromagnetic smog on the function of the autonomic nervous system by showing the decrease in heart rate variability through a technology called heart rate variability (HRV) analysis. A decrease in HRV is associated with autonomic nervous system dysfunction and, in turn, is associated with poor or deteriorating health. It also has been shown that electrosmog can change cell membrane's molecular sequences, affecting the critical functions of the cell membrane, which includes the effective intake of nutrients into the cell and the excretion of toxins and metabolic byproducts from the cell.

There has been a tremendous increase in the incidence of childhood and adult neurological and mitochondrial disorders in the last couple of decades, with electrosmog and mercury poisoning being major contributors. As a matter of fact, electrosmog may be the major cause of illness in children. Electrosmog also may be the main culprit behind the tremendous increase in mycotoxin concentrations in the human body. Mycotoxins are produced by mold and bacteria to protect themselves. With exposure to high levels of electrosmog at certain frequencies, there is a marked increase in the production of mycotoxins by these organisms in the body because of transformation of these organisms into much more virulent forms. That is one reason why we have seen such a dramatic rise in the incidence of fungal infections and a series of other infections, including Lyme disease, Chlamydia, Mycoplasma, Bartonella (the cause of cat scratch disease), Herpes, Epstein-Barr, and Cytomegalovirus infections. These

organisms contribute to some of the major illnesses of our time, including coronary heart disease, cancer, autoimmune diseases, such as rheumatoid arthritis and lupus, all kinds of neurological diseases, obesity, diabetes, chronic fatigue, fibromyalgia, and so on.

Neurological problems, including autism, ADHD, learning disorders, Tourette's syndrome, depression, and diseases associated with immune dysfunction, including a dramatic increase in the incidence of infections and autoimmune diseases, are becoming so common in our children that we are quickly reaching the point where no more normal children are being born. One of the reasons that this is happening is the fact that a fetus in the womb is the most vulnerable to electromagnetic smog and other toxins, like mercury. It is clear that genetic mutations also are occurring at a dramatically increased rate as a result of electrosmog. This is key in understanding the epidemics mentioned above. It is also noteworthy that many of these genetic mutations are brand new—in other words, not transmitted to the child by the parents. If no more normal children are being born, it means that we may not have enough normal people to keep our civilization going and therefore may be unable to continue the existence of the human race as we know it.

The good thing is that technologies already exist that can massively reduce EMF production, especially those producing the most harmful frequencies. There are also technologies and other things we can do that can reduce our exposure and limit the damage done. In those of us who are already damaged, there are some things that can mitigate the damage. We will review these solutions in the third part of this book.

Part II

The Roots of Illness and Pathway to Wellness

Unresolved Inner Conflicts and the Root Cause of Illness

Becoming aware of your life's story is a critical key to healing.

Maybe the most important discovery in medicine was made approximately thirty years ago by Dr. Ryke Hamer, the founder of "German New Medicine," when he came to the startling conclusion that cancer (and other illnesses) does not occur as random events. He discovered that diseases are programmed, biological events and are the expression in the body of unresolved conflicts.

He made this discovery after his own experience with cancer. He developed testicular cancer soon after his son died in 1978. Dr. Hamer, who was in his forties, unexpectedly lost his son, whom he loved dearly and was extremely close to. His son was murdered in what seemed to be a random violent act. The crime was never solved caused Dr. Hamer to experience profound psychological trauma that threw him into a deep depression that lasted for months. Soon after the depression lifted, he was diagnosed with testicular cancer. Dr. Hamer at the time had an intuition that the cancer diagnosis may have had something to do with his son's death and started putting a lot of thought into that possibility. He realized that when his son died, he himself had suffered a devastating, overwhelming loss that he was not prepared for that caused a massive unexpected shock to his system. He suspected that if he resolved this conflict and cleared the extraordinary emotional devastation that he had suffered, the cancer might resolve itself. This is exactly what happened.

During this period of severe inner conflict and prior to the diagnosis of his cancer, he had a series of symptoms, including severe insomnia, cold hands and feet, loss of appetite, severe mental fog, obsessive-compulsive thoughts about what happened, and other symptoms typically seen when humans go through severe stress. He was unable to concentrate, unable to work, and realized that he needed to come to terms with this loss if he was going to survive. With the support of friends, psychological counseling, and the love of his family, he finally turned the corner. Almost overnight he felt alive again, energetic and back on track in his life. Shortly after this, he felt a mass in his testicle and immediately had it evaluated by a colleague, who discovered the testicular cancer. Instead of chemotherapy, and radiation, Dr. Hamer decided to follow another path. He realized that this cancer had something to do with the psychological trauma he had experienced and the way he had processed it. He continued relentlessly to heal his psyche and a few weeks later, the cancer had resolved.

Dr. Hamer, the former head internist in the oncology clinic at Germany, at the time started evaluating every cancer patient he saw for a severe stressful event that preceded the cancer diagnosis and found that most of his cancer patients had had such an event within two years of the diagnosis, and all within ten years, and that the stress led to an unresolved psychological conflict that lasted a significant period of time at a high level. He also discovered that all those diagnosed with cancer felt isolated during their conflict and were unable to share their deep-seated feelings with anyone. They also had difficulty functioning in their everyday lives and had similar physical symptoms of stress.

Dr. Hamer also discovered that every one of them had a ring lesion in the brain visible on a CT scan corresponding with the body part or organ where the malignancy developed and that the nature of the unresolved conflict was very specific for the body part, organ, and type of cancer.

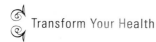

The Ways We Get Sick

A conflict initially occurs on a psychological level. As long as the conflict remains psychological, we remain healthy on a physical level; we become ill when the conflict becomes biological. Therefore, a biological conflict is an unresolved psychological conflict expressed in the body as a biological entity. When a conflict reaches a certain intensity where it threatens to overwhelm waking consciousness and the brain can no longer manage the body properly because of the amount of energy it is expending due to the psychological stress, it is pulled down into the body (into the biology). It is transposed by the brain in the area that corresponds to the exact tonality of the conflict; in other words, each part of the brain and each organ or tissue is impacted by specific conflicts and emotions.

Categories of Conflicts

A programming conflict creates the pathway in the brain and in the corresponding organ or tissue along which an illness can develop. In other words, it programs for a potential illness to develop either immediately or in the future. It often is incurred during childhood between the age of one and adolescence and occurs secondary to an emotionally traumatizing event.

A triggering conflict activates the pathway mentioned above and triggers the start of the evolution of an illness with the programming conflict analogous to a software program in place in the brain that gets launched by a second conflict that occurs sometime after the programming conflict.

Every physical illness is preceded by a programming and a triggering conflict. These can link up in different ways.

Programming and triggering conflicts occur together, triggering an illness. An illness can develop in an instant if the programming and triggering conflicts occur together; i.e., if the emotional or psychological shock behind the illness is overwhelming enough in intensity. For example, the loss of a loved one that we are emo-

tionally or physically dependent on may program for and trigger an illness at the same time. The requirement here is that the conflict is sudden, unexpected and overwhelms the waking consciousness to such a degree that it severely impairs day-to-day functioning. A good example would be Dr. Hamer's loss of his son discussed at the opening of this chapter and the association with his development of testicular cancer a few months later.

The programming conflict is followed later by a triggering conflict, fulminating in an illness. The premise here is that the programming and triggering conflict are of a similar nature, with the programming conflict occurring earlier in life. The programming conflict activates a biological pathway, which goes dormant before disease manifests to the point of being diagnosable. The triggering conflict that happens later reactivates this biological pathway, and diagnosable disease is the result.

For example, a mother nearly loses her son in a car accident when she is forty and her son is nineteen. He is admitted to an intensive care unit in critical condition, where he spends two weeks and ends up surviving and actually makes a full recovery. The woman notices discomfort in her left breast, plus a small lump a week or two later, but is consumed with taking care of her son, who takes a long time to recover (programming conflict related to a threat to her nest). She does not seek medical attention, but in spite of this, the discomfort and the lump disappear spontaneously a few weeks later. Six years later, she becomes estranged from her daughter, who is twenty-one at the time and disappears without a trace after a conflict with her mother. Eighteen months later, the daughter finds her peace and reunites with her mother (triggering conflict related to a threat to her nest). Two weeks later, the mother again feels discomfort in her left breast and again becomes aware of a lump. This time she sees her physician, who orders a mammogram and finds a suspicious-looking lesion, which turns out to be breast cancer.

An intense stress awakens old conflicts and triggers one or more diseases all at once. Here there are no similarities between the triggering conflict and previous programming conflicts, but the sever-

ity of the stress activates one or more dormant biological pathways associated with these previous programming conflicts. An example would be a gentleman who grows up very poor and then starts his own business, which becomes very successful. An employee then embezzles a large sum of money, forcing the owner to go bankrupt at age thirty-two (conflict of territory, with the business symbolizing his territory). He ends up starting over and again becomes successful. At age forty-eight, he falls victim to a robbery at gunpoint one night when he gets home late, with the assailant accosting him as he gets out of his car. The assailant flees the scene with the man's wallet and a couple of other items, but leaves him physically unscathed (conflict related to an immediate threat to survival). He ends up having a massive heart attack right in his driveway and passes away. The conflict of territory related to his loss of business at age thirty-two sets the biological pathway for coronary artery disease but does not lead to an event until an unrelated conflict of a very high intensity comes into play.

There are many other clues that are used to track these programming and triggering conflicts until the picture becomes crystal clear to the individual. These include extreme likes and dislikes, addictions, personality traits, phobias, and so on.

Deep High Stress (DHS): Dr. Hamer, through his own experience, had stumbled upon what he later called the "Dirk Hamer Syndrome," also called "Deep High Stress." He discovered the shock conflict mechanism underlying all cancer development and the development of disease in general (what he called cancer equivalent). There are certain unique characteristics of the shock that lead it to cause disease in the body.

1. First off, a conflict has to be dramatic to the point of overwhelming the senses and devastating the individual to the point where it becomes difficult to take action and to function in the normal sense. It can either be a single intense shock, as in Dr. Hamer's case, or it can be repetitive stresses that occur over long periods of time.

2. The shock also is normally unexpected and leads to a sense of defenselessness.

3. Another common characteristic of these traumas is that they leave the victim feeling isolated during the conflict and unable to share their feelings with anyone. The person affected is unable to communicate their deep emotions to others and ends up suppressing those emotions into the subconscious. This happens because he is either scared or embarrassed about communicating his innermost, overwhelming feelings, thinking that others might take exception or think that he is crazy. He also may feel that others are not reliable enough to share intimacies with.

4. Lastly, a characteristic of someone in this state of shock is a tendency toward obsessive thought about what has happened.

Like in this case, Dr. Hamer could not stop thinking about the perpetrator that had shot his son. He was in the position of massive sadness or feeling a tremendous sense of loss, and he just could not let go of it. He was literally thinking about it day and night, twenty-four seven, for a period of months. It was only when he realized that he was not able to function in this world anymore (if he continued on that track of extreme obsessive thinking that he was soon going to follow his son) that he was able to let go. As soon as he came to this realization, he woke up one morning feeling totally and completely at peace, as if a huge mountain had been lifted off his shoulders.

Breaker Switch Analogy

What Dr. Hamer also had discovered with this experience is something called the "breaker switch event." He started to realize that when we undergo a massive conflict like he did with his son's death, the stress to the brain becomes so overwhelming that it can suffer major damage in the same manner as a surge of high-voltage electricity can blow out the wiring in your home and cause a fire or a short circuit. In your home, there is a safety mechanism that prevents the frying of circuits; i.e., a breaker box with breaker switches that will trip when a surge of electricity occurs, thereby protecting your home against fire. The brain has a similar mechanism that, under circumstances such as major brain overload due to a high-stress event, will download the unresolved conflict associated with the overwhelming stress to a much smaller part of the brain, thereby protecting the rest of the brain from the potentially devastating surge of stress.

It's almost like a breaker switch in the brain. Once flipped, the emotional stress is downloaded in an instant to the smaller part of the brain. The DHS is also downloaded to the specific organ or part of the body that corresponds with a specific type of unresolved inner conflict (what Dr. Hamer called a biological invariant).

The Deep-felt Experience

The traumatizing events that we experience in our lives have very little to do with what happens to us health wise. It has far more to do with the nature of the inner experience of it; in other words, the deep-felt experience. How we experience a traumatic event depends on our interpretation of it. Our interpretation depends on a number of factors, including prior similar traumatic events. It also is based on our programming and belief systems, which stem primarily from the indoctrination by our parents, but also by other family members, friends, educators, clergy members, the media, politicians, and so on. Even our race, culture, and nationality play a potentially important role here.

We even carry memory imprints from our parents and other ancestors in our subconscious, which influence our interpretation of

potentially traumatic events. We call this epigenetic inheritance in contrast to genetic inheritance, which means that instead of it being in our genetic code, or DNA, we carry these memory imprints on our DNA, or cellular genetic code.

A conflict can be based on reality or imagination. It also can be virtual or symbolic in nature.

Conflicts based on reality result from actual traumatic experiences, i.e., your parents get divorced, and you experience a conflict of separation from one or both of them.

Conflicts based on imagination relate to circumstances where a traumatizing event has not taken place, yet the imagination can be so strong that it feels to the individual like the event has already happened. Even when a real trauma has occurred, a significant part of the experience may be imaginary. This is one explanation for the tremendous variation in eyewitness accounts of the same traumatic event witnessed by more than one individual.

A conflict is virtual in nature when the whole is represented by a smaller part or a minor aspect, i.e., someone was robbed at gunpoint in their kitchen while cooking pumpkin pie. Thereafter, every time the person smells an odor that reminds them of pumpkin pie, they become fearful of being attacked again or become panicky without remembering the connection between the odor and their previous trauma.

A conflict is symbolic in nature when a symbol represents a conflict; i.e., a burning cross is symbolic of right-wing extremist intimidation of blacks in the South.

The Nature of the Conflict
Defines the Type of Illness

The deep-felt experience resulting from a traumatizing event defines whether or not we get sick and what type of disease we might develop. Take the example of a wife who walks in on her husband while he is committing adultery with another woman. Any one of the following illnesses might result, depending on the nature of her deep-felt experience; in other words, the nature of the conflict that she experiences.

Leukemia—if she feels devastated, shamed, and devalued in relation to her family.

Coronary artery disease with a myocardial infarction (heart attack)—if she experiences it as a conflict of territory; i.e., another woman has invaded her territory, which includes her home and her husband.

Depression—if she feels devalued with a deep sense of guilt because she hasn't worked hard enough to please her husband to make him stay loyal to her.

Bladder problems—if she feels unable to mark her territory because of the presence of another woman in her territory.

Multiple sclerosis—if she feels devalued, feeling frozen (unable to move forward or backward at the sight of her husband in bed with another woman), and a fall from grace (symbolic of a vertical fall).

Colon cancer—if it's something she can't digest or get rid of, symbolic for being stuck in her gut.

No illness—if she is relieved because she has been attempting to find a good reason to leave him for a long time, or she has been unfaithful and now is able to come clean with no guilt because he is guilty of the same type of indiscretion.

Biological Invariant

A biological invariant refers to the correspondence between a specific conflict and a specific disease, meaning that a specific conflict will always trigger the same type of illness in any individual, regardless of race, culture, location, or situation—no exceptions.

The deep feeling, deep emotion at the moment of DHS determines: (1) The Hamer Herd; i.e., the specific targeted brain area (related to the targeted organ) and (2) the targeted body part and/or organ.

Specifically what this means is that each type of cancer or other disease that has been catalogued in the human race is related to a specific type of conflict, which downloads to a specific organ, part of that organ, or tissue. In the subsequent work that Dr. Hamer did, he discovered that even the area of the body, such as the breast, that is affected by a cancer, for example, is directly related to the nature of the conflict. He even discovered subtle variations in the unresolved conflicts that correlate with the specific part of the breast that is affected.

It also can be explained in the following way:

When an overwhelming stress or recurrent emotional stress is experienced in the conscious part of the brain, and if it threatens the survival of the individual by consuming too much of his concentration and his ability to be aware of his surrounding environment, it will download into the autonomic brain, which is directly associated with a certain body part, depending on the nature of the conflict. Once it downloads to the brain, it downloads to the associated body part at the same time. It was discovered by Dr. Hamer that in patients with cancer, there is a corresponding area of mild swelling in the brain, which he called a Hamer Herd. This lesion can be visualized on a (noncontrast) CT scan, for example, in every patient with a malignancy. Most radiologists call these lesions "artifacts"; in other words, they see them as meaningless and often don't even recognize them. These lesions are very subtle on CT scan, involve 1 percent or less of brain volume, and can only be seen by the trained eye of an individual who knows where to look and what to look for.

The location of the Hamer Herd always correlates with the specific nature of the conflict and the specific organ or tissue where the pathology is located.

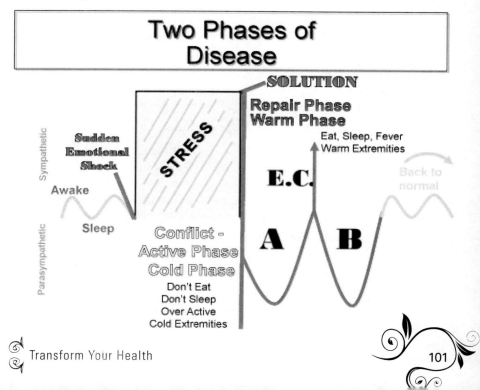

All Diseases Are Biphasic: Conflict Active Phase and the Resolution Phase

See page 138 for Chart

Every disease affecting the human body has two phases. In order to understand the pattern of any illness affecting the body, it is important to understand how each of these phases manifests as different facets of the disease.

In order to understand the two phases of illness, it is important to have a basic understanding of the autonomic nervous system. This is the part of the nervous system that acts automatically, controlling pulse rate, blood pressure, body temperature, blood flow patterns throughout the body, bowel and bladder function, and so forth. This part of the nervous system has two parts. The sympathetic nervous system and the parasympathetic nervous system, which have opposing, or "balancing," functions in every part of the body; i.e., the sympathetic nervous system increases heart rate and increases blood pressure, whereas the parasympathetic nervous system decreases heart rate and blood pressure.

The conflict active phase is triggered by an emotional trauma or shock, also called the DHS (deep high stress), and leads to the sympathetic nervous system going into overdrive, with symptoms typically associated with the "fight or flight response," which leads to a dramatic spike in the production of stress hormones, including adrenaline and cortisol. The symptoms associated with this phase include a sense of overwhelming, severe insomnia, cold hands and feet, a loss of appetite, severe problems concentrating and obsessive-compulsive thoughts about the event or situation responsible for triggering the DHS.

When no solution is found to alleviate the conflict that triggered the DHS, the conflict is downloaded to a smaller part of the brain (subconscious) and the body, with the resultant effects on the corresponding organ system or tissue, with the resultant disease often progressing imperceptibly outside the person's awareness.

The resolution phase, also called the healing or repair phase,

is initiated when a solution is found to the conflict, either through resolution or reframing. Conventional medicine can contain the physical aspects, even relieve the psychological impact, and can be life-saving. You heal (de-program the disease) only by finding and applying a solution to the conflict. The patient may not consciously be aware this has happened unless it was initiated through Recall Healing intervention or insight (the subject of Recall Healing will be presented in detail in Part 3). The sympathetic overdrive-related symptoms disappear almost instantly and are replaced by symptoms of parasympathetic nervous system dominance, including increased fatigue and increased need for sleep, warm hands and feet, hot flashes, increased sweating, fever, nausea and vomiting, increased appetite, headaches, dizziness, severe mental fog, physical weakness, and even short periods of paralysis.

The resolution phase has three subphases. The first subphase is called *post-conflictolysis phase A*, which starts at the moment the conflict is resolved. This phase is characterized as the brain repair phase, with swelling (edema) occurring in the brain in the region of the zone of neurons involved in the disease phase (Hamer Herd). This occurs as a result of blood flow normalizing to this region, bringing oxygen and other nutrients to help in the healing process. This localized swelling in the brain may compress surrounding brain tissue, leading to symptoms like headache, dizziness, brain fog, nausea, and vomiting.

The second subphase is called the *epileptoid crisis*, which lasts for a few hours to a day and is characterized by a sudden reoccurence of the symptoms present during the conflict active phase. This subphase occurs when enough healing has taken place in the Hamer Herd area of the brain to turn its functions back on again, switching from disease (survival) program back to normal function in that part of the brain (breaker switch in the brain turns back on again). This is also the phase where seizures may occur, depending on the disease program launched prior to the healing phase.

The third subphase is called *post-conflictolysis phase B*, or the restitution phase, during which the affected organ or tissue in the body

starts healing. This phase usually occurs rather rapidly and often is associated with symptoms specific for that organ or tissue involved in the initial download during the conflict active phase. Scarring may result, depending on the intensity of the conflict and the disease load carried in that organ or tissue. A scar also typically remains in the brain at the center of the Hamer Herd previously present. If a similar conflict occurs in the future, the body will recreate the same pathology in the brain and the body with great efficiency as a result.

Two Basic Disease Patterns

Every disease falls into one of two basic disease patterns and one of four basic subpatterns, and is controlled by the brain, which launches the disease program in the first place.

1. Brain signals for increase.

a. Increased cell division (cell proliferation)

In certain organs and tissues, the brain signals for increased cell division, leading to the forming of a mass. This happens during the conflict active phase, resulting in a polyp, cyst, fibroma, tumor (benign or malignant; i.e., adenocarcinoma of the breast, prostate, and so on) or a general increase in tissue; i.e., increase in fat cells in obesity.

During the resolution phase, the brain signal for increased cell division is nullified, leading to reversal or reduction of the mass with the aid of organisms such as mycobacteria and fungi.

b. Increased function

Here the brain signals for the increase of function in certain organs or tissues or the unblocking of certain functions again during the conflict active phase, leading to conditions such as hyperthyroidism (increased thyroid hormone production), tremors (i.e., intention tremor or Parkinson's), Tourette's disorder, and so on. During the resolution phase, functions return back to normal or near normal.

2. Brain signals for decrease.

a. Decreased cell division

Transform Your Life

Here the brain signals for cellular reduction in certain organs or tissues, leading to increased porosity (i.e., osteoporosis), ulceration (i.e., in the nose mucous membrane just before a cold occurs, or skin just before the onset of eczema), or destruction (i.e., cartilage destruction during osteoarthritis). During the resolution phase, cell division increases, leading to repair of porosity, ulcerations, destruction often with the involvement of organisms such as viruses and bacteria, leading to conditions like bone tumors (bone porosity repair), leukemia (bone marrow repair), common cold (nasal mucous membrane repair), myocardial infarction (repair of inner lining of the blood vessels), and so on.

b. Decreased function

Here the brain signals for the decrease of function in certain organs or tissues or the unblocking of certain functions again during the conflict active phase, leading to conditions such as hypothyroidism (low thyroid production), diabetes, multiple sclerosis, myopia (nearsightedness), and so on. During the restoration phase, function increases back to normal or near normal and the reversal of conditions such as those mentioned above.

The Nature of the Conflict Defines the Nature and Location of the Disease

In Dr. Hamer's case, the conflict that he went through when his son died was "conflict related to loss of a child," which in normal biological terms in the animal kingdom would simply lead to further procreation. In the human species, this is somewhat more complex, but the primitive biology of our brains still expresses conflicts in the body just as it has for eons. So when Dr. Hamer had lost his son, in his testicles, during the conflict active phase, there was a process of ulceration (enlargement) of the seminal tubes in the testicles that continued during the months that Dr. Hamer was going through his conflict before it resolved. The biological intent of this ulceration process is to prepare the testicles to store more sperm so that

the animal (or human being) can procreate rapidly after the threat is resolved. During the recovery phase (resolution phase) from the conflict, the ulceration in the seminal tubes resolves rapidly as the body attempts to heal these ulcerations through cell division and cell proliferation (cells multiply). In the testicles, it is during the healing phase that the tumor develops as a result of initial over compensation with some excess in cell proliferation. The body overshoots during the resolution phase, especially following a DHS event. This would normally be followed by reabsorption of cells and a reduction or disappearance of the mass in the testicle, unless a second conflict comes into play or unless the initial conflict failed to resolve fully.

Disease Linked to Embryonic Layers

Every disease results from pathological changes in organs or tissues. Every organ or tissue originates from one of three embryonic layers that form during the first three weeks of fetal development and is directly linked to a specific control center located in one of four regions in the brain.

Every disease is a biological program that originates from a Deep High Stress (DHS), which is a conflict or shock that downloads simultaneously to the psyche, a specific location in the brain, and a specific organ or tissue. The specific location in the brain and organ or tissue depends on the specific nature and tonality of the conflict or shock.

Exactly what happens in the organ or tissue is defined by the embryonic layer that the organ/tissue originated from during fetal development and which phase the disease cycle is in; i.e., conflict active phase or conflict resolution phase.

Every infection occurs during the conflict resolution phase, is part of the healing process, and actually accelerates healing through tissue modulation and can get out of hand and even cause death. The type of organism is defined by the embryonic layer that the tissue or organ originated from.

The three embryonic layers that form very soon after conception

include the endoderm, mesoderm (which includes the old meso-derm and the new mesoderm), and ectoderm. The four brain regions and organs that originate from them, the effect on tissue during the conflict active phase (sympathicotonia—S phase), the effect on tissue during the conflict resolution phase (Vagotonia—V phase), the microbes associated with each embryonic layer, brain region, and associated organs, as well as the categories of conflicts/shocks that download to them are summarized in the following paragraphs.

The *endoderm* gives rise to the brain stem and key vital organs, including the gastro intestinal tract, liver, kidneys, pancreas, and the sex organs. A mass forms during the S phase (conflict active phase), and during the V phase (conflict resolution or healing phase), the growth of the mass stops and the mass becomes encapsulated or is destroyed by fungus or mycobacteria. The categories of conflicts or shocks that download to the brainstem and its associated organs include morsel (either can't take in food or something symbolic of food or nutrition or can't excrete feces or urine or something symbolic of feces or urine), abandonment, existence, or refugee conflicts.

The *old mesoderm* gives rise to the cerebellum part of the brain as well as the deeper layer of the skin (dermis), the protective membrane around the lungs (pleura), the protective membrane around the abdominal cavity (peritoneum), the protective membrane around the heart (pericardium), and the protective membrane around the brain (meninges). Like with the endoderm and its related organs, a mass forms during the S phase (conflict active phase), and during the V phase (conflict resolution phase), the growth of the mass stops and becomes encapsulated or is destroyed by fungus, bacteria, or mycobacteria. The categories of conflicts or shocks that download to the cerebellum and its associated organs include conflicts relate to protection (i.e. feeling under threat of an attack which can be real, imaginary or symbolic) and conflicts related to nurturing or feeding.

The *new mesoderm* gives rise to the cerebral medulla (the white substance of the brain) as well as bones, muscle, and connective tissue, which includes tendons, ligaments, and the subcutaneous tis-

Transform Your Health

sues underneath the skin. Tissue death or ulceration occurs during the S phase (conflict active phase), and during the V phase (conflict resolution phase), regeneration or reconstruction of destroyed tissues take place. A mass or cyst may form, and scar formation can take place due to healing of ulcerated tissue or areas of tissue death. The microbes that are involved in conflict resolution phase include bacteria and viruses. The categories of conflicts or shocks that download to the cerebral medulla and its associated organs include conflicts related to value and production or productivity (devaluation), loss, stand (my ability to stand or symbolic i.e. my standing) and conflicts related to movement like walking and running.

The *ectoderm* gives rise to the cortex (the grey substance of the brain cortex), the surface layer of the skin (the epidermis), the nervous system, the inner layers of the blood vessels, the bladder, the larynx, the cervix, and the rectum, as well as parts of the testicles and ovaries. Like with the mesoderm and its related organs tissue death or ulceration occurs during the S phase (conflict active phase), and during the V phase (conflict resolution phase), regeneration or reconstruction of destroyed tissues take place. A mass or cyst may form, and scar formation can take place due to healing of ulcerated tissue or areas of tissue death. The microbes that are involved in the conflict resolution phase again includes bacteria and viruses. The categories of conflicts or shocks that download to the cerebral cortex and its associated organs include conflicts related to separation (relational), territory (territorial), laterality, and our relationship with the outside world in general.

Conflict of the Diagnosis and Prognosis

Once the tumor is felt by an individual, another switch is triggered in the brain called a "diagnosis or prognosis switch." Initially, that is related to self-diagnosis, and with an expanding awareness of cancer and an expanding tendency toward fear of cancer whenever a tumor or a mass is felt by most people, the brain will attempt to figure out

the nature of the problem. And as a part of the survival mechanism, the brain will tend to consider the worst possible threats first.

For example, as in nature, when the brain hears a roar, it has to decide if that roar is a giant lion coming toward a helpless victim or a helpless cat at the top of the tree. So, when a tumor is first brought to the awareness of an individual, either through self-awareness or diagnosis from a scan, a mammogram, or another test, the brain immediately adds an additional massive conflict phase called the "conflict of the diagnosis or prognosis." This internal conflict load gets dramatically worse and might even change in nature; i.e., a conflict related to the fear of death can compound a conflict of the nest like in certain breast cancers with the conflict of the fear of death, downloading as a lung cancer, complicating the breast cancer.

This conflict of the diagnosis or prognosis escalates exponentially when a firm diagnosis of cancer is made, often confirming the worst fears of the individual being examined. This leads to the secondary conflict download from the brain, which cannot handle overwhelming stress and worry associated with a diagnosis such as cancer and downloads it further into the body, often to a secondary area, where it results into a secondary malignancy, which is almost always mistaken by Western medicine for metastatic cancer originating from the original cancer.

So, when a woman develops breast cancer, it triggers a massive diagnosis or prognosis conflict within her and she develops an intense fear of death. If the fear of death persists for a certain length of time at a certain volume of intensity, that particular conflict will download as a lung metastasis. The unresolved conflict linked to lung cancer is the fear of death. It's no wonder that most metastases are to the lung (conflict related to the fear of death) or liver (conflict related to the fear of starvation—the need to store extra nutrients in case the cancer shuts off the GI tract and prevents the human from being able to eat).

Dr. Hamer was so bold as to state that the conflict of the diagnosis or prognosis embodies about 90 percent of the disease load in the body and 99.9 percent of exacerbations. This is an extraordinary

discovery because if you look at what is happening in our society, you see that we are becoming more and more cancer-conscious. There is more and more fear of cancer, so it is natural that when a diagnosis of cancer is made and shared with an individual, the subconscious not only takes on the personal fears of the person diagnosed, but also the fear linked to mass consciousness related to that diagnosis. That is one of the great downsides of our knowledge revolution.

Having information about problems, diseases, and maladies without having information on solutions is a very dangerous thing. In many ways, it's better not to know that you might be sick from a biological perspective than it is to know that you are dealing with a potentially life-threatening illness with either no good solutions or solutions with potentially devastating side effects, like mutilating surgery, chemotherapy, or radiation therapy. Of course, in our world today, there has not been a practical solution because of the fear of litigation that physicians deal with. This often leads them to be extremely thorough in communicating all possible negative outcomes of the disease and the side effects of possible treatments so that if that outcome happens, they have done their due diligence and warned the patient of the possible outcome. They don't want to be liable for any problems that occur.

How ironic that the legal profession has complicated medicine in such a huge way because of our fear of litigation. Again, unfortunately, the fact is that we live in a very reactive society that tends to look for the "quick fix" instead of the "deep fix." We have great difficulty as a society focusing on what is in the highest interests of the individual in our society. If it were not so, we would be able to revolutionize the treatment of cancer and other diseases overnight.

Three Layers of Downloads

We also need to be aware that all diseases follow natural biological laws. When we are born into this world, we are not empty vessels, as most would like to believe, but come pre-programmed with lots of data and programs that are meant to enhance the likelihood of

Transform Your Life

our survival and that have been carried in the memory banks of our forbearers for many generations. This means that some of the health challenges that we deal with need to be tracked further back than the conflicts of a single individual's lifetime. What it means is that we often have to go back on a practical level (as far back as four generations) to understand what has been downloaded to the afflicted individual who is presenting with an illness or disease.

In Recall Healing, we look at no fewer than three layers of downloads that can lead to illness.

The first layer includes those traumatizing events that take place starting about the first year of life through the present that lead to programming conflicts, further aggravated subsequently by triggering conflicts. This was discussed earlier in this chapter.

The second layer of downloads and the second major source of biological conflict, your project purpose, is set by one year of age and comes directly from your biological parents. Every person has a purpose that corresponds to the project that was made for it by its creator; i.e., the biological parents. This programming is linked to the period starting nine months before conception through to our first year of life. This is another survival tool and is essential for the parents to be able to function at a level in this world where they have the greatest chance of being able to support their offspring and continue to procreate.

The unresolved psychological conflicts of the parents become the biological conflicts of the child. For example, if a women becomes pregnant in order to "keep her man" because of stress in the relationship, the child conceived will carry the conflict of "keeping mommy and daddy together." Later on in life, if there is discord between the mother and the father, or if they get divorced, the child's subconscious conflict will escalate to the degree where he may become physically ill with an illness representative of the conflict of separation, like eczema.

Even factors like how your parents felt about becoming pregnant with you and what exactly the nature of their conflicts were at the very time of your conception manifest as downloads and become

part of your underlying operating principles that set the tone for your life. Of course, most are unaware of this until they start digging deeper in order to heal.

Let's look at another example: If a woman becomes pregnant, and the father is absolutely livid (angry) about the pregnancy and disappears out of the mother's life shortly after he gets word that she is pregnant, even if the mother is at peace and wants the baby, that child will come in with an intense conflict related to feeling unwanted. This is even worse when both parents do not want the child. If the mother doesn't want the baby, even if she changes her mind after the first three months, the stage is already set for that child to come into this world feeling he's not likely to please anyone no matter how hard he tries. He will always invite rejection and hardship in his life.

On the other hand, when the pregnancy is welcomed and both parents are ecstatic throughout the pregnancy, that baby will tend to come into this world feeling wanted, especially if this environment remains stable for at least the first year after birth. No matter what that child does in life, he'll tend to have pretty good self-esteem and self-respect. This is one great explanation of why some people come into the world with an incessant lack of self-confidence, self-esteem and self-respect and no matter what they achieve in their lives they constantly keep striving for more and more. They never feel like they make it, while others seem to be a lot more at peace.

The third layer of downloads we receive when we come into this world are downloads related to our genealogy and the transfer of family memories from one generation to another going back as far as four generations. Here, birth order becomes critical because what has been noticed by those studying this phenomenon is the fact that a concept called "biological cascades" exists.

Our birth order—in other words, our numerical position in our family clan—determines which ancestors are linked to us vertically and horizontally. If you are a firstborn, for example, you are aligned with other number ones, but also with fourth, seventh, and tenth-born family members. Second-born family members align

Transform Your Life

with other second, fifth, eighth, and eleventh-born family members; third-born family members with other third, sixth, ninth, and twelfth-born, and so on. In order to establish an accurate birth order, every pregnancy should be counted, including those that ended prematurely, as in miscarriages, abortions, and stillbirths.

Some of the important characteristics that are often shared between family members that are in genealogical alignment include issues like key struggles, personality strengths and weaknesses or shortcomings, manner of death of those deceased, diseases, professions, and especially family secrets—the unspoken issues in the family—that contribute a great deal to the biological conflicts of subsequent generations.

Biological Cascades

One of the laws of emotional and biological inheritance reads as follows:

The manifestations of each person in each generation of their respective family clan are always the expression of the circulating memories in biological cascades, indefinitely until resolution of the conflict. At that moment, the descendants are set free.

What does that mean? It means in a family where territorial conflicts have existed for generations, the generations to come will tend to experience and literally play out the same dramas, leading to the same conflicts. Let's look at the case of a thirty-five-year-old man (we will call him Ed) who dies of a massive heart attack and leaves his family devastated and perplexed at his sudden departure. When revealing Ed's history, it is discovered that just prior to his massive heart attack, he had gone though a massive conflict related to loss of territory.

What had happened is that Ed had gone into business with a friend (we'll call him Joe) after years of very hard work on a new idea. Ed had a great talent for detailed work in terms of innovation and creation of new things. Joe had a different set of talents that dovetailed and complemented Ed's talents very nicely. As a matter

of fact, Joe's talents included being a great promoter and seller, and he was certainly comfortable with small and large crowds and did a great job promoting those projects that Ed was responsible for creating and making. One day, Joe did something quite underhanded and decided that the company would do much better if he was in charge of it. Through trickery, he got his partner, Ed, to sign off on a contract, unwittingly giving full control of the company to Joe.

Ed had the habit of going through the motions of signing off on hundreds of documents as CEO and as creator in this company. He was not a detailed-oriented person and did not like to read the small details in everything that he signed. He believed the people around him were taking good care of him, and he could trust them fully and completely, knowing that they had gone through the details of each piece of paper they needed him to sign. As it turns out, Ed was wrong about Joe, and basically, he was pushed out of his own company. Instantly, he went through a massive conflict related to territory. Ed fought tooth and nail to get his company back. He hired lawyers and spent a small fortune, but did not prevail. After the final battle was fought and he could do no more to get his company back, within twenty-four hours, he was dead from a massive heart attack.

What was surprising is that Ed's last twenty-four hours were wonderful! He had gone through tremendous turmoil, and relief had finally struck as he came to terms with the loss of his company and made peace. Then he suffered a massive heart attack (myocardial infarction).

It is important to note that myocardial infarctions always occur during the conflict resolution phase and are linked to a conflict of territory. It is also noteworthy that if the territorial conflict is of very high intensity and if the conflict active phase lasts eight months or more, the likelihood of a catastrophic fatal MI is very high.

In the case of this man (Ed) dying of a heart attack, it is interesting to note that when you go back into his family history, you find that his father died at age fifty-seven (also of a heart attack) after a similar conflict of territory tragedy. The story details are different, but the nature of the story was very similar. His father had lost

Transform Your Life

everything at a time in his life when he felt that he was making great progress and had gone through a natural disaster in a place that he lived. An earthquake struck his home and business. After the loss of his home and his business, he subsequently lost his wife (who left him after twenty-two years of marriage because she just couldn't deal with having to start all over again with nothing), and more devastation occurred. At the time of the tragedies, they did not have insurance on his business. They had worked hard as immigrants to make it in this country. Going back another generation, the father had an uncle who also died of a heart attack and who was in the same birth order as he (also born third just like the father was). The uncle also suffered a massive conflict of territory. While growing up in Europe, he was pushed aside by two older siblings when it came to dividing up his parents' estate, which was very large at the time. The father of the uncle had died relatively young (in his forties) and had left millions of dollars to his children. The two older sons, who were much more business-savvy, figured out how to cheat the third child out of his inheritance. The third child, after he became an adult, fought as hard as he could to get his inheritance back, but at that time was unsuccessful because of the connections that the two other brothers had in the town that they lived in and the fact that no judge or politician would go up against these two brothers. That child subsequently became an older man, went through another tragedy relating to territory (a triggering conflict) later in life, and passed away of a massive heart attack soon after (at approximately sixty-three years of age). So here is a case of a biological cascade starting with the third-born uncle to his third-born nephew and then a direct download from the third-born nephew to his son (Ed).

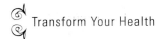

A Historical Perspective on Epidemics

This point is further illustrated by an extraordinary piece of our recent history. In 2005, when hurricane Katrina destroyed a big part of New Orleans, approximately two thousand people died during the flooding caused by the hurricane. But the part of the story that's never been covered by the media is the part that speaks to the true magnitude of the effects of biological laws and the effects on health.

In the aftermath of Katrina, when tens of thousands of people started straying back toward New Orleans to go and see what had happened to their homes and to gather what little belongings remained (in many cases, nothing existed), an extraordinary thing happened. In case after case, people would get to the place where their homes used to be and no longer were, or would stand in front of their devastated or condemned houses and would have heart attacks on the spot or soon after. For so many who had to leave New Orleans in the aftermath of Katrina, they had to deal with the conflict of loss of territory (their homes), sometimes for many weeks before they were able to get back to see their homes. Some of them even took months before they were able to get back to see, either because they did not have proper transportation to get back or just were in severe reaction mode and were scared of what they would see.

Seeing their destroyed homes was like a relief from a biological perspective. When you fear something and when you have intense emotional stress related to something, when it comes to fruition or when you see the full manifestation of it, it literally creates relief. In other words, the biological solution for the fear of something is the occurrence of that something, which then allows you to move on.

Again, it is fascinating to note that biological conflicts don't just affect the individual, but sometimes masses of people. For example, during the Second World War in Europe, a massive epidemic of tuberculosis occurred soon after the war came to a conclusion. When the Germans surrendered in 1945, a massive number of people started coming down with tuberculosis all across Europe, with all kinds of measures taken to get the epidemic under control. Again,

the fascinating thing about tuberculosis (and also of lung cancer) is that the underlying conflict of the disease is the fear of imminent death of self or of loved ones, and tuberculosis always occurs during the healing phase of this conflict.

Across Europe there was a mass fear of death that resulted from the constant bombing back and forth between the Germans and the countries in Europe that were allied against Germany. When the conflict ceased, there was massive relief all across Europe, leading to "conflict resolution" of this mass fear of death. During that conflict resolution, it is not strange at all, then, that tuberculosis broke out because the tuberculosis bacterium, or the organism that causes tuberculosis, actually flourishes in the aftermath of this biological conflict, as the bronchial tubes of the lungs start to heal from the ulcerations of the bronchial tubes linked to the conflict active phase. In other words, during a conflict of fear of imminent death, the lungs will do everything in its power to expand the volume to get more air by creating ulceration of the inner layers of the bronchial tubes. When that conflict of the lung (the fear of death) resolves, it leads to the recovery of the mucous membrane and an over-proliferation of the cells of the mucous membrane, leading to tumor formation as a result of overcorrection from the ulceration, leading to narrowing of the bronchial tubes. The mycobacterium that causes tuberculosis is actually involved in the healing phase, causing the destruction of these tumors in the lung.

The reason why tuberculosis has almost disappeared in Western Europe is because of the low fear of imminent death, brought about by political stability, low violent crime, and low fatal accident rates over the past fifty years or so.

When you look into all of the plagues of history you will find that there was a common underlying societal conflict at the time that set the stage for that particular epidemic. The type of organism involved, either virus or bacteria, has everything to do with the type of conflict, the intensity, and the nature of the conflict.

It is not the bug that makes us sick; it's the vulnerable host that

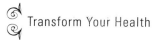

gets sick. What makes the host vulnerable to the infection is primarily dependent on the type of biological conflict that has just resolved and the organ or tissue it is linked with. How we infect each other by sharing organisms doesn't have to do with the organism itself being infectious as much as it has to do with an unconscious sharing of inner conflicts. If you look at the common cold or flu, if there is a communication breakdown in a group of people and an unconscious conflict of no communication comes into play, that will lead to the group as a whole becoming more vulnerable to flu or a cold. In other words, even the organisms involved in our illnesses are part of the biological solution implied with every unresolved inner conflict. In summary, it's not the bug that makes you sick. It's the vulnerable host, in the healing phase following a significant inner conflict, with the organism related to the healing phase and specific to the tissue type and its relationship to the part of the brain that originally downloaded into the body.

Summary of the Biological Laws Governing Illness

The discoveries made by Dr. Ryke Hamer boil down to the fact that biological conflicts, which are unresolved conflicts expressed in the body as biological entities, form the root cause of all illnesses. He also discovered the existence of biological laws that apply 100 percent of the time in terms of the development of disease. Dr. Claude Sabbah, a French physician who founded "Total Biology," expanded on Dr. Hamer's work and made some other key discoveries that shed further light on the biological laws that govern disease formation and healing through conflict discovery and resolution. Dr. Sabbah in his almost thirty years of research and practice also has stated that he has never identified a single case of illness that does not obey these natural biological laws.

The main factor in illness is not your genes, nor is it diet or

toxicity or infectious organisms, even though they play a peripheral role. All these factors, though, have one thing in common: they are all linked to these same biological laws. The disease program itself launched by the brain in response to a deep-felt conflict directs the role and impact of other factors, such as those mentioned above. We will expand on this later.

To summarize some of the biological laws discovered by Dr. Hamer, he found the following principles to be true:

1. The brain is the central control station, and illness is a program that the brain can switch on under circumstances of extreme stress or a very significant conflict experienced by a living creature.

   Disease is the brain's best solution to keep the person alive as long as possible. Therefore, disease is a survival program. The brain is like an electric device, and the disease is one of its programs, which is switched on in specific circumstances of high stress or conflict and switched off when the high or prolonged stress or conflict is released or resolved!
   —Claude Sabbah

   The brain can switch off this same illness-creating program as soon as the conflict that triggered the creature's illness has been resolved or is eliminated.

2. There is a consistent and profound link between the symbolism of illnesses, the part of the body that is affected, and the corresponding parts of the brain.

3. Every so-called disease has to be understood as a "meaningful, special biological program of nature" created to solve an unexpected, biological conflict. Disease, therefore, is not a fault, but an adaptation.

Healing depends on identifying and removing the source of conflict within.

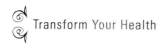

Dr. Claude Sabbah stated, "To heal from any illness, it is necessary and sufficient to remove the source of conflict within oneself."

What Dr. Hamer discovered next was most startling, and that is, when the unresolved conflict was discovered and resolved, 95 percent to 98 percent of his patients got better. These are extraordinary results in a field where cure rates are a far cry from these kinds of numbers, and the treatments themselves are typically very harmful in their own right and contribute a great deal to high complication and death rates.

The patients treated by Dr. Hamer who failed to heal had one or more of the following three factors in common.

1.   The primary conflict was still unresolved. There was still an aspect of the unresolved conflict that had not been identified or cleared. This was very unusual for Dr. Hamer not to be able to discover or help clear his patient's primary conflict. This is more common for those practitioners with less experience or proficiency than Dr. Hamer, and their success rates are therefore lower to a greater or lesser extent.

2.   A major secondary conflict had developed after the diagnosis of cancer was shared with them in a way that traumatized them further. He called this the conflict of the diagnosis or prognosis. In other words, if the patient had a great fear of death resulting from the way the diagnosis was conveyed or based on their view of cancer or the experience of family members with cancer, then the result was further expansion of the cancer and often the development of metastatic disease. For example, with an intense fear of death, a second cancer would develop in the lungs. In orthodox medicine, metastatic cancer is always blamed on the original cancer, but Dr. Hamer and others have found that the exact nature and type of cells of the lung metastasis are different from the original tumor in most cases.

Transform Your Life

3. A third category would include those who had reached the point of no return. In other words, their disease was so advanced at the time they were first seen that it had already caused sufficient compromise in the major organ systems to prevent or curtail the body's ability to heal itself. In other words, death becomes the biological solution. You can read more on this later.

The Iceberg Analogy in Recall Healing

When you see an iceberg floating in the ocean, what you are really seeing represents less than 10 percent of its total mass. What is even more fascinating is what you see is not even real because of how the top of the iceberg reflects in the water. You only realize this when you get up close to it. Our personal realities are similar because what we are aware of in our individual universes amounts to less than 10 percent of reality, that part that we can perceive through our five senses. Not only do we perceive less than 10 percent of reality but also this perception is by and large completely false. True reality has very little to do with superficial appearance. It is important not to remain in the world of appearances, on the surface of things.

To find true reality, one needs to go deeper, beyond the surface. In order to understand this concept even better, it helps to gain at least a rudimentary understanding of the laws of quantum physics, which govern the subatomic sphere of existence and by extension the macroscopic sphere as well. Our biological brain is connected with the true reality of the universe.

Often we become victims of knowledge, seeing that most knowledge is based on false reality. On the other hand, true knowledge liberates. We may be embarrassed with or overwhelmed by a disease, but for biology, disease is an asset (a solution)! We need to learn how to see reality as it truly is by using a different approach; i.e., by considering every dimension of being human.

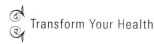 

Shadows in the Mind

Most of humanity is totally unaware of what you are reading about in this chapter. The conflicts at the root of our diseases are invisible to us, like a shadow in the mind or a "blind spot." When a conflict threatens to overwhelm the brain and is downloaded to a smaller portion of itself and to the body, it also disappears from our waking consciousness. It disappears into the subconscious, where it remains until it is searched for and discovered, all the while affecting your health. This happens as a critical adaptation to enhance the chances of short-term survival. Dr. Claude Sabbah coined the term "mini-maxi schizophrenia" to describe this phenomenon. Schizophrenia occurs when we totally lose track of reality and are immersed in an imaginary world. A mini-maxi schizophrenia implies that we are steeped in reality except for our downloaded conflicts, which disappear from waking consciousness, but are often clearly visible and discernible within us by close friends and family.

Disease Is Related to Survival Programming

At a biological level, we all carry survival programming corresponding with the entire hierarchy of living things, reaching from the very bottom of the evolutionary ladder to the very top. Imagine an inverted pyramid with all animals at the top, all vertebral animals second, all mammals third, all primates fourth, all humans fifth, your family next, and you last. In the world of creatures (human, animals, plant, and so on), every living thing is programmed to survive as long as possible at any cost. So every biological modification (disease, health, and so on) has a profound meaning. We may be overwhelmed or embarrassed because of a disease, but for nature this is, at least over the short term, a winning program. Over the medium-to long-term, the disease itself becomes counterproductive, leading to disability and sometimes even death.

Disease is the brain's best solution to keep the organism alive as long as possible. Every disease represents the biological correspondence between the organ that is sick, the part of the brain that controls that organ, and the specific biological conflict at the level of the psyche (mind, thoughts, feelings, and so on) that programs for the disease. So in summary the mind analyzes, the brain commands, and the body executes the specific biological conflict programming for a specific illness or disease.

We will be discussing some of the ways in which conflicts can be resolved in order to set the stage for possible miraculous healing in part three.

For additional information on the subject of Recall Healing, go to www.academyCIM.com for online courses on Recall Healing taught by Gilbert Renaud, PhD and David Holt, D.O., H.M.D Also visit Gilbert Renaud's Web site recallhealing.com for information on his Recall Healing seminars given around the country.

The Anatomy of an Illness

In the previous chapter, we discussed the fact that disease is a biological solution to unresolved inner conflict. It is the brain's best solution to keep the body alive.

On a physical level, a second phenomenon takes place in which the body becomes ill. The psychological conflict affects the energy field in a particular region of the body, as described in the previous chapter. When the energy field is weakened, it sets the stage for the trapping of toxins and the proliferation of infectious agents in a particular part of the body. It also can be explained in another way, which is that when an unresolved inner conflict weakens the energy field in a particular region of the body, that part of the body is unable to eliminate toxins and infectious agents, therefore allowing an accumulation of those agents to take place. The regions and types of tissues involved are conflict specific and emotion specific.

Homotoxicology

Another term used in the study of toxicity in the human body is "homotoxicology." Homotoxicology is a theory of disease developed by Dr. Hans-Heinrich Reckeweg (1905–1985) that understands illness as the human body's defense against toxic substances that threaten to overwhelm those defenses. According to this arm of medical science, the type and severity of an illness is determined by the duration and intensity of toxin loading in relationship to the body's inherent capacity for detoxification.

In homotoxicology, the term "matrix" is used to describe the spaces in between the cells. Most people think of the body as a conglomeration of cells, with blood vessels, bones, and tendons somewhere in the mix. What is important to realize, though, is that the matrix makes up a large part of the body and has within it an intricate network of structural collagen fibers, tiny blood vessels, nerve fibers and something called ground substance. This matrix is critical to the health of the human body because it's through this space that nutrients move from the blood vessels to the cells, and toxins move from the cells to the lymphatic system and the blood vessels. Clogging of this matrix obstructs the movement of nutrients and toxins to and from the cells, disrupting the natural balance in the body and hindering critical biological processes. The resulting disturbances, which eventually manifest as illness, are the body's attempt to restore a state of internal harmony (biochemical balance). To Dr. Reckeweg, the whole purpose of medicine and all medical treatments should be to restore balance.

Homotoxicology as a healing modality is one of medicine's great success stories. It also has been completely ignored by conventional medicine. Originally conceived to explain the incredible efficacy of a distinct path of homeopathic medications, this model of treatment has grown into a comprehensive theory of disease that helps to create a road map from disease to wellness.

The Disease Evolution Table

The disease evolution table (see page 133 and 137), first developed by Dr. Reckeweg and later expanded to include more details, is a diagrammatic representation of a coordinated system showing the relationship between the degree of clogging in the intercellular matrix and possible health consequences. The table's six columns show increasing toxin loads (on the horizontal axis) in relationship to the disturbances they cause in different organs (on the vertical axis). Progression of a patient's illness (called progressive vicariation) is tracked from left to right, whereas improvement (regressive

Transform Your Health

vicariation) is tracked from right to left. When the body is exposed to toxins, the body defends itself and protects itself in a very predictable manner along the hierarchy of organ systems and through different phases representing distinct detox and defense mechanisms. The hierarchy of organ systems is based on the idea that toxicity proceeds into the body progressively through different systems, starting with those that are least essential for the maintenance of life to those that are most essential. Roughly speaking, toxins tend to migrate from the outside in and from the top down. When the body heals, it tends to heal in a reverse order, from the bottom up and from the inside out.

Six Phases of Disease Evolution

There are six phases of disease evolution with three overarching phases represented on the horizontal axis. These phases represent the body's defense mechanism and how toxins invade from the periphery to the center. It starts with the humoral phases, whereby the body reacts by activating excretion mechanisms and where inflammation sets in. This process is followed by the matrix phases (spaces between the cells but outside the blood vessels), where more deep-seated damage occurs and where reversal (regressive vicariation) is progressively harder to achieve without outside help, such as anti-homotoxic therapy. In the cellular phases, actual cell damage becomes evident, starting from the periphery of the cell and ending with damage to the cell nucleus and the genetic code (DNA). Damage in the cellular phases is very hard to reverse without extraordinary support measures and if too far advanced may be nearly impossible. In other words, there is a point of no return, beyond which the organ and oftentimes the body as a whole start shutting down. The current version of the Disease Evolution Table in this book includes the most frequently encountered diagnosis.

Let's take the nose as a relatively simple, but representative, example. When a toxin (or infectious agent) enters the nose and settles on the mucous membrane, the body under normal circumstances will rid itself of this offending agent through its normal

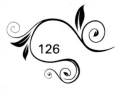

Transform Your Life

defense mechanisms, which include mucus formation, the sweeping action of microscopic ciliary hair, and an occasional sneeze. If the toxin is present at levels that threaten to overwhelm the natural defenses either because of the amount of toxicity or because of a compromised defense system, the body will attempt to boost the activity of these nasal defense mechanisms.

The initial response will be for the mucous membranes in the nose to attempt to excrete the toxin (*excretory phase*). Increased mucous production is the result, with a runny nose as the main symptom. If the nose is successful in excreting the toxin, it will regain normality. However, if it is unable to excrete the toxin efficiently, then the next homotoxicology phase will kick in.

During this phase, the mucous membrane gets inflamed. The individual will start sneezing excessively, and the nose may start itching (*inflammatory phase*). Again, if successful, reversal will take place to the previous phase, and a runny nose will complete the job. However, if that defense mechanism is overwhelmed, it will go to the next phase (*deposition phase*), with the spaces in between cells now involved. Again, in an effort to protect itself, the mucous membrane in the nose swells up in order to increase the distance that toxins will have to travel before deeper tissue can be invaded. The symptoms experienced would be congestion or stuffy nose.

In order to illustrate the total 180-degree difference in the approach of conventional medicine compared to natural, integrative, and holistic medicine, we can look at the nose and these three phases and how differently they are treated and the consequences that we can expect.

Conventional medicine and more specifically the pharmaceutical industry prides itself on creating an ever-expanding list of drugs for the treatment of every imaginable symptom of disease. We have just learned, however, that symptoms are indicators or reflections of the body's defense mechanisms in action. So, when someone has a runny nose, conventional doctors prescribe decongestants or drying agents, e.g., antihistamines for sneezing and itching and steroids or steroid nasal sprays for congestion or swelling of the mucous mem-

brane. The competence of conventional doctors is measured based on how effective they are at suppressing symptoms, but almost no attention is paid to the long-term consequences of these symptom-suppression strategies. Physicians who prescribe the most drugs are the favorites of the pharmaceutical industry.

Look closely because herein lies the seed of discontent. When a symptom is treated effectively, the treatment tends to paralyze the very defense mechanisms in the body that are desperately attempting to keep the toxin from penetrating deeper into the body and further down along the hierarchy of organ systems. Remember, the hierarchy of organ systems goes from least essential for life to most essential for life. Skin, for example, is at the top, whereas the immune system is at the bottom and most essential for life. When you open a gateway that facilitates the penetration of toxins deeper into the matrix and into the cells, you are inviting disaster.

Let's continue on our journey through the nose. We have reached the *deposition phase* with swelling of the nasal mucous membranes, beyond which the biological division line is reached. This biological division line represents the threshold beyond which the organ moves from inflammation in a general sense (first three phases), where the organ or system attempts to rid itself of toxins, to containment, where the body tries to cordon off the toxic load to prevent it from affecting more critical functions and organs in the body. The three containment phases to the right of the biological division line move the organ or system toward degeneration and eventually to dedifferentiation.

If the nasal mucous membrane is able to contain its exposure to toxins and stays to the left of this biological division line, healing is relatively straightforward, because all that has to be done is to bolster the defense mechanism and reduce toxin exposure so it can complete its mission to recover successfully. The therapeutic goal should, therefore, be to support the body's defenses rather than break them down. When the right treatment is used, paradoxically, we may notice a brief spike in symptoms. For example, if the nose is currently in the inflammatory phase, and sneezing and itching are

Transform Your Life

occurring and the right homeopathic remedy is administered, the patient may briefly start sneezing more, and then will move back into excretion phase with an increase in excretions from the nose moving progressively toward normalcy.

When the biological division line is crossed, we enter the domain of the degenerative phases. The first phase to the right of the biological division line is called the *impregnation phase*. In the example of the nasal mucous membranes, generalized swelling gives way to the formation of masses like polyps, which are benign in nature and are still clearly identifiable as mucous membrane. These polyps form in an effort to contain the toxins that have now invaded to this level. These masses also may start affecting the bony structure and cartilage in the nose, and the nose may look more bulky and swollen. In conventional medicine, we have now reached a point of no return, where the only solution is either to administer higher doses of steroids to get some reduction in swelling, or to do surgery to remove the polyps. The problem with administering steroids, for example, by nasal spray is that it leads to chronic sinus infections caused by fungal organisms due to the weakening of local defenses against fungal invasion. In studies done at Mayo Clinic, it was shown that a fungus was responsible for 96 percent of the cases of chronic sinusitis.

Continuing the journey through the nose, we see that when toxins go beyond the matrix and start invading the cells, cells start becoming dysfunctional and eventually lose their function or die. The nasal mucous membrane enters the *degenerative phase* and is eventually unrecognizable as mucous membrane and incapable of performing the functions of normal mucous membrane. It becomes more like dry parchment than luscious, moist, warming, humidifying mucous membrane. So what to do now? Conventional medicine has very little, if anything, to offer at this stage to help relieve symptoms. Patients often are prescribed more steroid sprays for discomfort, such as severe nasal dryness, which further accelerate degenerative changes.

So what happens when invasion reaches the core of the cell?

Again, either cell death occurs, or the genetic code becomes so defective that malignancies may occur. This phase is called the *dedifferentiation phase*, and if malignant transformation is the result, treatment in conventional medicine usually involves surgical removal of the tumor and surrounding tissue and may include radiation therapy and chemotherapy. Reversal of this phase and the previous degenerative phase is still possible, but much harder to achieve.

Vertical Invasion through the Hierarchy of Organ Systems

In addition, invasion of toxins does not just happen on the horizontal level, but also vertically. So when we destroy the body's ability to defend itself in one organ system, toxins will start affecting the next organ system down the line. For example, toxicity and infectious organisms affecting the respiratory tract (sinuses or lungs) may jump to the next level of organ systems down—i.e., the cardiovascular system—then to the urogenital system, and so forth until the immune system is reached. By the time the immune system has been totally incapacitated, life becomes impossible to maintain.

Another Disaster in the Making: Treating High Cholesterol

Expanding on the example of toxicity and infectious organisms moving from the respiratory system to the cardiovascular system, here is another good demonstration of how conventional medicine contributes to disease formation when the focus is on controlling a symptom, like high cholesterol levels. We now know, based on dozens of studies, that inflammation of the inner lining of the blood vessels constitutes the greatest risk factor for the development of coronary artery diseases, fulminating in a myocardial infarction (heart attack). Cholesterol, which receives most of the blame, actu-

130

Transform Your Life

ally plays a minor role in its development, whereas inflammation of the inner lining of blood vessels plays a far greater role.

Cholesterol, in fact, is a molecule that is vital to health and is a critical component of every cell membrane in the human body. It is also the basic building block of a large number of hormones in the human body, including the adrenal and sex hormones. The liver produces most of the cholesterol found in the human body, with less than 15 percent coming from the foods we eat. When the liver is stressed, it produces more cholesterol in order to protect itself and to help repair damage to tissues elsewhere in the body. It is true that the aggressive treatment of cholesterol reduces the incidence of myocardial infarctions, but not because of reduced cholesterol levels, but because the most commonly used drugs, the statin drugs, actually reduce inflammation in blood vessels. The lives saved by preventing heart attacks come at a great price. By treating cholesterol as the enemy, conventional medicine is contributing to a number of other disease epidemics by dramatically weakening the body's ability to protect against the invasion of toxins to deeper levels (progressive vicariation). The body cannot exist without cholesterol, and because of the very aggressive treatment of cholesterol in those at risk for coronary artery disease, we are seeing a dramatic increase in the incidence of conditions like heart failure, depression, memory problems, impotence, liver problems, muscle weakness, decreased stamina, chronic fatigue, and more.

Scientists have been tracking the incidence of congestive heart failure, and there seems to be almost a perfect match between the increasing incidence of congestive heart failure and the increasing number of prescriptions for statin drugs. This also happens to be the most profitable group of drugs in the history of the pharmaceutical industry.

One of the reasons why more and more physicians and scientists are convinced that there is a connection between the statin drugs and congestive heart failure as well as decreased stamina and muscle weakness is because the statin drugs are known to impact dramatically on the production and/or levels of coenzyme Q10. Coenzyme

Q10 plays a critical role as far as intracellular energy production. This is especially important in tissues like the heart muscle, where cells produce and use a lot of energy. The statin drugs tend to reduce this intracellular energy production, eventually leading to a progressive weakening of the heart muscle and an increased risk of congestive heart failure. Yet, in spite of this knowledge, the vast majority of physicians don't even recommend that patients taking these drugs also take coenzyme Q10.

Bolstering Defenses: A Far Better Approach to Healing

I hope it is now abundantly clear how dangerous it is to interfere with the body's defense mechanisms by taking pharmaceuticals blindly and how important it is to do everything in our power to bolster the body's defenses and also to reduce the toxin load. If you are involved in a serious accident and need to be put back together again or have a severe overwhelming infection of any kind, you are a candidate for the most powerful drugs that conventional medicine has to offer. If your blood pressure is through the roof and threatening to cause a stroke or heart failure, then you want the best antihypertensive drugs medicine has to offer, at least over the short term. If your blood sugar is sky high and you are in imminent danger of kidney failure or blindness as a result, then you want the best drugs that conventional medicine has to offer. However, if you just keep taking drugs, you may be doomed to more and more misery as your body spirals through the layers and phases of disease as described in the Disease Evolution Table.

DISEASE
EVOLUTION
TABLE
(DET)

and

Two Phases
of Disease

DISEASE EVOLUTION TABLE (DET)

HEALTH ← Status of Regulation / Deregulation

			Humoral Phases	Matrix Phases
Organ System/Tissue		**Excretion Phase**	**Inflammation Phase**	**Deposition Phase**

ECTODERMAL

Organ System/Tissue	Excretion Phase	Inflammation Phase	Deposition Phase
1. EPIDERMAL	Increased sweating, Cerumen, Sebum, Smegma	Dermatitis, Impetigo, Abscess, Furuncle, Otitis externa	Hyperkeratosis, Seborrhoic eczema, Naevus, Skin tags (soft warts)
2. ORODERMAL	Hypersalivation, Hyperlacrimation	Otitis media, Pharyngitis, Stomatitis, Gingivitis, Apthous ulceration, Glossitis, Rhinitis (acute), Sinusitis (acute), Laryngitis, Dental abscess	Nasal polyp, Eustachian tube catarrh (serous otitis media), Dental granuloma
3. NEURODERMAL PNS and CNS	Increased secretion of neurotransmitters	Neuralgia, Neuritis, Polyneuritis, Meningitis, Encephalitis, Trigeminal neuralgia (acute)	Neuroma, Amyloid deposition, Heavy metal deposition
4. EYE		Conjunctivitis (acute)	Pterygium, Mouches volantes (floaters), Iris spots (initial)
5. SYMPATHICODERMAL	Increased adrenalin and noradrenaline secretion	Flushes, Hypervagotony, Hypersympathicotonus	Ganglion neuroma

ENDODERMAL

6. MUCODERMAL

	Excretion Phase	Inflammation Phase	Deposition Phase
1. Respiratory	Sputum	Bronchitis (acute), Tracheitis	Nasal polyp
2. Digestive	Increased digestive juices	Esophagitis (acute), Gastritis (acute), Gastroenteritis (acute), Colitis	Gastric polyps, Intestinal polyps, Obstipation, Melanosis of the colon
3. Urogenital	Increased mucous production	Bartholinitis, Cystitis, Urethritis, Infections of the urogenital mucosa	Bladder polyps, Uterine polyps

7. ORGANODERMAL

	Excretion Phase	Inflammation Phase	Deposition Phase
1. Exocrine Sexual	Lactorrhea	Mastitis	Mammary cysts, Breast calcifications
2. Exocrine Digestive	Increased bile salt secretion, Increased gastric acid secretion	Pancreatitis, Sialitis	Cholelithiasis, Steatosis hepatica, Pancreatic calcifications, Pancreatic cysts, Liver cysts, Wilson's disease, Salivary gland calcifications
3. Respiratory		Acute pulmonary abscess, Pneumonia	Bronchiectasis, Pneumoconiosis
4. Endocrine	Increased thyroid hormones, Parathyroid hormones, Thymic hormones, Insulin, Glucagon, Enteric hormones, Cortico-suprarenal hormones, Adenohypophyseal hormones	Thyroiditis, e.g. de Quervain's thyroiditis	Thyroid cysts, Adrenal cysts, Adrenal adenoma, Hypophyseal adenoma, Thymoma, Insulinoma, Parathyroid gland adenoma, Thyroid goiter, Adrenal adenomas

see rest of graph on the following pages

Transform Your Life

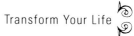

DISEASE EVOLUTION TABLE (DET)

Status of Regulation / Deregulation ➔ **DISEASE**

Matrix Phases   Cellular Phases

Regulation/Compensation	Impregnation Phase	Degeneration Phase	Dedifferentiation Phase
	Atopic eczema, Urticaria, Warts, Fissura ani, Acne rosacea, Hirsutism	Psoriasis, Decubitus ulceration, Radiation injury, Pemphigus vulgaris	Squamous cell carcinoma, Basal cell carcinoma, Melanoma
	Atopic rhinitis, Hay fever, Sinusitis (chronic), Rhinitis (iatrogenic), Anosmia, Menière's syndrome, Hypoacusis	Otosclerosis, Deafness (transmission), Ozaena, Atrophic rhinitis, Dental caries, Parodontosis	Leucoplakia (orodermal), Cancer of the tongue, Laryngeal cancer, Nasopharyngeal cancer, Tracheal cancer
	Epilepsy (petit mal), Paresis, Tics, Neuritis (toxic), Attention-deficit/hyperactivity syndrome (ADHS), Guillain-Barré syndrome, Poliomyelitis (acute), Trigeminal neuralgia (chronic)	Parkinson disease, Epilepsy (grand mal), Alzheimer's disease, Multiple sclerosis, Amyotrophic lateral sclerosis, Peripheral neural atrophy, Diabetic neuropathy, Neurofibromatosis	Glioma, Meningioma, Astrocytoma
	Uveitis, Allergic conjunctivitis, Iris spots (chronic), Iritis, Astigmatism, Myopia, Presbyopia, Keratoconus, Pannus, Arch (senile)	Glaucoma, Cataract, Hemianopsia, Macular degeneration, Paralytic mydriasis	Retinal cancer, Retinoblastoma
	Dysautonomia (including orthostatic hypotension)	Addison's disease, Reflex sympathetic dystrophy (RSD) or Sudeck's syndrome, Horner's syndrome	Pheochromocytoma, Neuroblastoma
	Bronchitis (asthmatic), Chronic tracheitis (viral), Cystic fibrosis	COPD (chronic obstructive pulmonary disease), Atrophy of bronchial mucosa	Tracheal cancer, Bronchial cancer
	Gastric ulcer, Duodenal ulcer, Gluten enteropathy (mild), Leaky gut syndrome, Dysbiosis	Crohn´s disease, Colitis ulcerosa, Atrophy of the small intestinal villi, Gluten enteropathy (severe)	Barret's esophagus, Esophageal cancer, Gastric cancer, Duodenal cancer, Rectal cancer
	Interstitial cystitis	Atrophy of the urogenital mucosa	Bladder cancer, Cervical carcinoma
	Mammary fibroadenoma, Fibrocystic mastopathy	Breast atrophy, Gynecomastia	Mammary carcinoma
	Chronic hepatitis, Chronic pancreatitis, Viral pancreatitis (e.g. mumps), Alcoholic hepatitis, Cystic fibrosis	Hepatic cirrhosis, Hepatic iatrogenic disease	Liver cancer, Pancreatic cancer
	Bronchial asthma, Cystic fibrosis	Emphysema, Chronic pulmonary abscess, Interstitial fibrosis of the lung, Fungal balls	Pulmonary cancer
	Grave's disease, Hashimoto's disease (1st stage), Puerpural thyroiditis, Cushing's syndrome, Precocious puberty, Adrenal exhaustion	Hashimoto's disease (2nd stage), Riedel's thyroiditis, Parathyroid atrophy	Thyroid cancer, Parathyroid cancer, Adrenal cancer, Carcinoid syndrome

see rest of graph on the following pages

Transform Your Health

DISEASE EVOLUTION TABLE (DET)

HEALTH ⬅ Status of Regulation / Deregulation

		Humoral Phases		Matrix Phases
8. CONNECT. TISSUE		Increased secretion of metalloproteinases, Increase in glycoprotein formation	Abscess, Reactive inflammatory response of the matrix, Tendinitis	Lipoma, Storage of toxins in the matrix, Amyloidosis, Mucopolysaccharidosis, Periarthritis humeroscapularis calcinosa
9. OSTEODERMAL			Osteomyelitis, Chondroitis	Osteophyte formation, Bone cysts
10. HEMODERMAL	1. Blood		Leukocytosis neutrophila, Anemia related to acute infection	Thrombocytosis, Polycytemia (reactive), Hypercoagulation
	2. Heart	Increased cardiac output, Tachycardia	Myocarditis, Extrasystoles, Acute rheumatic fever	Left ventricular hypertrophy, Coronary atheroma
	3. Vascular	Increased production of endothelial mediators	Phlebitis, Arteritis, Endothelial inflammation	Venous stasis, Arterial plaques (atheroma), Hemorrhoids
11. LYMPHODERMAL		Increased lymph production	Tonsillitis, Adenitis, Adenoiditis, Lymphangitis	Lymph edema, Lymph adenopathy, Tonsillar hypertrophy, Adenoid hypertrophy
12. CAVODERMAL		Increased synovial liquid, Cerebrospinal fluid	Arthritis, Polyarthritis, Synovitis, Acute rheumatic disease	Hydrops (articular), Gouty tophi, Hemarthrosis
13. NEPHRODERMAL		Frequent urination	Nephritis, Glomerulonephritis, Pyelitis	Nephrolithiasis, Renal cysts, Renal sand, Orthostatic albuminuria, Hematuria
14. SERODERMAL		Increased production of serous fluid	Pleuritis, Peritonitis, Pericarditis	Pleural effusion
15. GERMINODERMAL	M Increased seminal fluid		Prostatitis, Epididymitis, Orchitis	Spermatocoele, Early benign prostatic hyperplasia (BPH)
	F Heavy menstruation		Ovaritis, Adnexitis, Metritis, Dysmenorrhea	Ovarian cysts, Uterine polyps, Uterine fibroids
16. MUSCULODERMAL		Myalgia	Myositis	Myogelosis, Myositis ossificans

MESODERMAL

MESENCHYMAL

Regulation/Compensation

Self regulation. | **Self-healing effects.** | **Favourable Prognosis.**

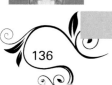

136

Transform Your Life

DISEASE EVOLUTION TABLE (DET)

Status of Regulation / Deregulation ➡️ **DISEASE**

Matrix Phases   Cellular Phases

Regulation/Compensation	Matrix Phases	Cellular Phases	
	Mixed connective tissue disease (MCTD), Marfan's syndrome, Ehlers-Danlos syndrome, Sphingolipidosis	Scleroderma, Carbohydrate deficient glycoprotein syndrome, Peyronie's disease, Progeria, Dupuytren's contracture	Sarcoma
	Osteomalacia, Early osteoporosis	Osteoporosis, Paget's disease	Osteosarcoma
	Eosinophilia, Leukopenia, Anemia (including anemia of chronic disorders), Hypercoagulation	Aplastic anemia, Thrombocytopenia (including idiopathic thrombocyopaenic purpura), Pancytopenia, Vaquez's disease	Leukemia
	Angina pectoris, Atrial enlargement, Arrhytmia cordis, Rheumatic fever affecting the heart, Prolapse of the mitral valve (Barlow's syndrome), Cardiomyopathy	Myocardial infarct, Ventricular arrhytmia, Stenosis and insufficiency of the cardiac valves	Sarcoma
	Vasculitis, Arteriosclerosis, Varicose veins, Panarteritis nodosa, Angioma, Varicocele	Peripheral vascular disease, Aneurysm, Arteritis obliterans	Angiosarcoma
	Indurated edema, Venerial lymphogranuloma, Cat scratch disease	Lymphatic tuberculosis, Elephantiasis	Lymphoma (Hodgkin's, Non Hodgkin's), Lymphosarcoma
	Chronic arthritis, Reiter's syndrome, Hydrocephaly, Spinal disc herniation	Arthrosis, Ankylosing spondylitis	Sarcoma, Chondrosarcoma
	Pre-clinical nephrosis, Nephrotic syndrome, Chronic hematuria, Goodpasture's syndrome, Auto-immune glomerulonephritis	Nephrosis, Chronic glomerulonephritis, Tuberculosis of the urogenital tract	Hypernephroma, Wilms' tumor
	Chronic exsudative pleuritis and serositis, Ascites, Chronic pericarditis	Pleural, pericardial and peritoneal tuberculosis, Pleural adhesions	Mesothelioma, Primary peritoneal carcinoma, Primary pleural cancer
	Benign prostatic hyperplasia (BPH), Oligo asthenospermia	Sterility	Prostate cancer, Testicular cancer, Seminoma, Teratoma
	Chronic adnexitis, Amenorrhea	Infertility, Ovarian atrophy	Ovarial cancer, Ovarial teratoma
	Muscular asthenia, Mitochondrial myopathy, Autoimmune dermatomyositis	Muscular atrophy, Muscular dystrophy	Myosarcoma

Compensation.   **Tendency to aggravation.**   **Doubtful Prognosis.**

Printed with permission of the International Academy for Homotoxicology GmbH

Transform Your Health

Two Phases of Disease

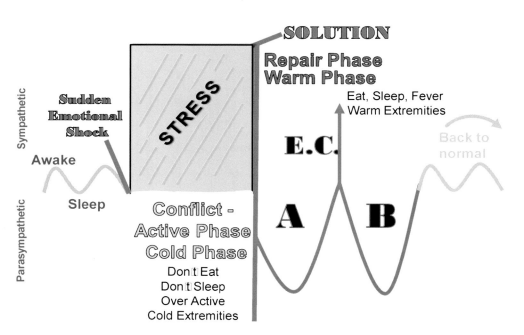

Printed with permission of Gilbert Renaud, PhD

Transform Your Life

The Five Levels of Healing

There are too many natural healing modalities available today to list or describe here in this section, but the common denominator among all of them is the bolstering of the body's own defense mechanisms and the activation of the body's own healing systems guided by an inner intelligence that is capable of bringing about miraculous healing even in the presence of advanced or life-threatening illness.

Ancient writings from India dating back approximately ten thousand years describe a healing system that makes tremendous sense when attempting to navigate your way through the maze of healing modalities available to us today. The five levels of healing are based on the five bodies described in the ancient Yoga Sutras, written by Patanjali, an Indian Master. Dr. Dietrich Klinghardt, MD, PhD, who is one of the world's leading authorities and instructors on advanced natural healing systems, through his contemporary interpretation of this ancient healing system has made it a lot easier for anyone to understand the basic principles of effective healing, including how one might induce one's own healing.

I want to make the point that even though this book is about self-healing, it should be clear to each of us that taking responsibility for one's own healing doesn't mean that you should do it all without any assistance. In order to heal, we all need support from family and friends. We all could benefit from having cheerleaders and coaches to help us stay on track and to learn new skills and sharpen others to help us be successful in our healing endeavors. Yes, and most, if not all, of us should seek help from qualified health professionals at

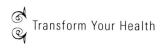

times in order to figure out what might be wrong or what healing modalities might be helpful in our quest for overcoming disease and optimizing health.

An important point that needs to be made, and one that Dr. Klinghardt emphasizes, is that healing can only be effective long-term if we heal at the level at which an illness was triggered or at levels above that. If we work at levels below that, we can at best expect temporary and incomplete healing, no improvement, or at worst continued or even more rapid progression of disease.

It is also important to note that each higher level has an organizing influence on lower levels, which means that healing on level four, for example, will tend to bring about the reorganization and healing at the next level down, and so forth. Healing at the higher levels often brings about rapid, sometimes even instantaneous healing at the lower levels. It is necessary, however, to work on the lower levels in order to provide the physical energy for healing at higher levels.

There are five levels of healing. They include the physical body (level 1), energy body (level 2), mental body (level 3), intuitive body (level 4), and spirit body (level5).

Physical Body

The physical body is, of course, that part of us that can be perceived by the five senses. This is the level of structure and biochemistry. At this level, issues such as misalignments of spinal vertebrae or other joints can contribute to illness. It is also at this level that nutritional deficiencies and toxins play an often-critical role in making us ill.

Tools used for diagnostic purposes at this level include a physical examination, blood work, microscopic evaluations (such as in pathology), genetic testing, and autonomic response testing (applied kinesiology, also called muscle testing).

Healing modalities that apply to this level include pharmaceuticals, which we already mentioned typically target symptoms of disease and not the root issues. Other modalities include nutritional

Transform Your Life

therapies, such as; diet, vitamins, minerals, enzymes, other nutritional supplements, hormones, herbs, aromatherapy, and homeopathics at lower dilutions. Detoxification strategies and the treatment of nutritional deficiencies are key components of healing at level one. Surgery, colonics, chiropractic and osteopathic manipulation, physical therapy, massage, and exercise also belong to this level. Eliminating structural misalignments is also very important for regaining health.

Energy Body

This level is the level linked to physics and physiology. The physical body is surrounded and penetrated by an energy field, which consists of electromagnetic, gravitational, weak nuclear and strong nuclear forces, as well as light emissions. The electromagnetic force is linked to the electromagnetic charge that every living cell carries and especially the flow of electrical energy along the nerve fibers traversing the human body. The body also is surrounded by a bio-photon field (light field), which is linked to photons (light emissions) released by every living cell, especially the DNA in the nucleus of the cell. This field plays a critical role in the communication between cells throughout the body. Each of these forces can be measured by modern scientific devices. Our feelings and emotions also are linked to this level.

This level is affected by a variety of modern technologies which are contributing tremendously to the ill health of us as individuals and to society as a whole. Devices such as cordless phones, Wi-Fi systems, electrical devices and wiring in our homes, microwave ovens, cell phones, and cell phone towers have some of the most devastating effects. Read the chapter on electromagnetic smog for more information. Irradiation due to nuclear contamination, X-ray radiation from diagnostic devices, light pollution, and scars on the body affecting meridian energy flow also come into play on this level.

A wide array of technologies used in modern medicine, both diagnostic and therapeutic, operates at this level. This includes

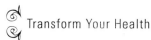

x-rays, magnetic resonance imaging, electrocardiograms, electro-acupuncture by Voll devices (bioenergetic diagnostic devices), heart rate variability, thermography, and many others. Autonomic response testing (applied kinesiology) is also very helpful in the evaluation of problems at this level, as well as levels 3 and 4.

Therapeutic modalities at this level include a number of energy medicine tools, such as healing touch, Reiki, acupuncture, electro-acupuncture, microcurrent therapies, and activities such as Yoga, meditation, and Qi Gong. Neural therapy; mesotherapy; segment therapy; and scar therapy, often with the use of procaine, a local anesthetic with remarkable healing properties, are some additional tools used to reset the autonomic nervous system and the electromagnetic charges on cells in general where dysfunction is occurring. Homeopathics at medium dilutions, including flower remedies, are also very helpful at this level because they are able to treat negative emotions at the physiological, hormonal, and neurological level.

Mental Body

This level is linked to our belief systems, thoughts, feelings, and perceptions, which, in turn, organize our emotions and other aspects of the energy body. This body is both individualized and at the same time linked to and influenced by mass consciousness or consensus reality. Unresolved psychological conflicts (feelings buried alive) stemming from the traumatic experiences of our lives affect us at this level and form the root of most illnesses, especially when you add to that the conflicts we inherit through our genealogy and the conflicts we take on that relate to mass consciousness (level 4). The role of unresolved conflicts in the development of disease is laid out in greater detail in the first chapter of this part of the book. Erroneous belief systems also form a key component that leads to dysfunction at this level.

Evaluation tools here include those used in Recall Healing, which involves taking a history with a focus on past events and traumas, which programmed for disease, analysis of belief systems, psy-

142

choanalysis, and psychokinesiology (autonomic response testing to evaluate the subconscious).

Healing modalities that apply to this level include homeopathics at higher dilutions, such as flower remedies, which work at levels 2 and 3. Other modalities include Recall Healing (works on levels 3 and 4—see the first chapter of this part); German New Medicine (pioneered by Dr. Ryke Hamer); Total Biology (pioneered by Dr. Claude Sabbah; works on levels 3 and 4); Evox voice analysis related to self, personal beliefs, and personally experienced emotional traumas; psychological interventions, such as psychotherapy, hypnotherapy, timeline therapy, gestalt therapy, and emotional freedom technique (EFT), which combines level 3 (psychological reprogramming) with level 2 (tapping on a series of acupressure points); mental field therapy (also works on levels 2 and 3); and applied psychoneurobiology (pioneered by Dr. Dietrich Klinghardt, which combines a number of modalities listed above and works on levels 3 and 4).

Intuitive Body

This level relates to the collective unconscious, also called mass consciousness. Not only do we carry our own individual unresolved conflicts, but we also carry the conflicts of our genealogy, our cultures, ethnicity, races, our communities, religions and even of humanity as a whole. The most important conflicts to track down relate to our genealogy going back four generations, including us. Any conflicts that led to a loss of love, respect or intimacy need to be tracked down, if possible. Also critical is to acknowledge and bring to light family secrets and to heal the wounds left by devastating losses of loved ones in past generations.

Healing modalities that apply at this level include Recall Healing, Total Biology, Evox voice analysis related to parents and other family members, applied psychoneurobiology, systematic family constellations, hypnotherapy, color and sound therapy and shamanism. A critical goal of healing at this level should be the reestablishment of love and respect in the family and the assimilation and recognition of all members of the family going back at least three generations. It should include the identification and the lifting of the veil on toxic secrets carried in the family. Healing at level 4 often brings about instant healing at level 3 with the instant healing of unresolved personal conflicts downloaded to the brain and to the body as disease.

Spirit Body

This is the level of religion and spirituality and the level of self-healing. One must overcome spiritual destitution in order to create an overarching framework for healing. This level of healing requires us to go within in order to connect with our Creator and our divine essence, the ultimate source of healing. This is the level of unconditional love, ecstasy, unbridled joy of being, inner peace despite our health situation or life circumstances, and a feeling of oneness with all and oneness with our Creator, of enlightenment and pure consciousness. If this is achieved, then healing is profound and automatic. It requires, however, the transcendence of the ego, relinquishing judgment and righteousness, and dualistic and other erroneous beliefs.

Gratitude is one of the most effective tools in healing and is required for the purpose of healing at this level. This includes gratitude for adversity, infirmity, antagonism, and anything else life might throw at us. Prayer and affirmations can be extraordinarily effective tools for healing. Studies on prayer have shown that not only does it work to relieve the suffering of those who are prayed for, but also of those doing the praying for others. Selfless giving (altruism) has also been shown to correlate with a much greater likelihood of good health and healing. Shifting the focus from self to assisting others is another critical key to healing on this level.

Erroneous Belief Systems

Do our beliefs and the way we look at ourselves and our universe contribute to suffering and the development of health problems? The answer is, *Yes!* As a matter of fact, you could say that the root of all suffering can be found in our thoughts and our beliefs. Suffering is not related to what we go through. It is related to our point of view; in other words, how we interpret our experiences. Our interpretation of our experiences, in turn, is related to our frame of mind, which is based on our beliefs.

The Source of Our Beliefs

Our beliefs stem from the totality of experiences of our lives and how we interpret those experiences, and the experiences of our parents and how they interpreted them, and what we are indoctrinated with and domesticated with from birth on. The vast majority of our beliefs are inherited. The programming of our beliefs starts at a subconscious level from the moment of conception. During the gestational period in the womb and after birth to approximately one year of age, we continue to be programmed by literally absorbing the unresolved psychological conflicts, deep-felt emotions, and strongly held beliefs of our parents into the subconscious. There also appears to be epigenetic transfers of unresolved conflicts and deeply held beliefs from our genealogy to the individual that takes place at conception. Even if your maternal grandmother died while she was giving birth to your mother, because your mom spent the first nine

months of her existence in your maternal grandmother's womb, your mother will possess many of your maternal grandmother's emotions and beliefs, which your mother could have passed along to you when you were in her womb.

Conscious programming takes place starting from approximately age one, when awareness of us as individuals starts taking place. By seven years old, the personality is pretty much fully developed and set, with the domestication process playing a critical role. From age seven through fourteen, development of the imagination is at the forefront, with a very strong focus on feelings. From age fourteen to twenty-one, development of the higher mind and intellect takes place. We start seeking our own identity apart from our families and start developing our independent power of judgment and decision making.

We are programmed primarily based on the beliefs of our parents or primary caregivers, as well as other family members, friends, television and the media in general, our teachers, religious figures, and so forth. There is some additional programming that takes place after age fourteen, but this is relatively small, at less than 5 percent. In other words, 95 percent of our deeply held beliefs are programmed by age fourteen.

Our past experiences and how those were interpreted, our personality traits, the genealogical downloads from our parents and other immediate ancestors, and mass consciousness or group consciousness all also play a key role in forming our belief systems. Again, suffering is not defined by what happens to us, but by how we interpret those experiences, which is based almost entirely on our beliefs. Following are a few key examples.

Suffering Versus Ecstasy

Is it possible for two people to go through the same situation and have different experiences? Let's look at a couple of examples. Two people go on a roller-coaster ride sitting right next to each other, going through the same ups and downs, sudden acceleration and deceleration, similar physiological responses with bursts of adrenaline,

accelerated heart rate, hollow feeling in the stomach, tension in the muscles, and so forth. They go through the same physical experience in real time but may have totally different interpretations. One may be exhilarated and ecstatic and want to go right back to do it again and again. The other may be scared out of her wits and may never want to do that again. Their deep-felt experience is totally different.

In many of the great religions of the world, for example, you will find that what others see as suffering is often incorporated in many of the rituals, whether it is fasting leading to hunger, self-isolation leading to the pain of separation or the infliction of physical pain. In Thailand, Buddhist monks often perform rituals that involve lying on beds of nails, walking on shattered glass with their bare feet, the penetration of the skin with sharp barbs, and so on. The deep-felt experience that the typical participant in religious rituals like these has is totally opposite of what someone would experience if these same acts or circumstances were forced upon him. The difference is primarily based on their differing underlying beliefs about what they experience, which defines the nature of the deep-felt experience.

Death: In the Eye of the Beholder

Even the way we look at death depends totally on our belief systems. In most Western cultures, death is seen as the enemy that needs to be defeated or delayed as long as possible at any cost. A morbid fear of death is very common in our society even though most people, for example, in the United States are religious and believe in life after death.

In many Eastern cultures, death is celebrated because of their belief in reincarnation. They believe that when you die, you will return to earth again and again in a cycle of reincarnations, with each incarnation bringing you closer to escaping the cycle to a higher reality or dimension. The focus tends to be on building good karma during your life to ensure progression of the soul to better incarnations. In some of the most radical sects of certain religions, not only is death celebrated, but terminating the lives of as many infidels (nonbelievers) as possible while terminating your own—i.e., the suicide bomber—is embraced and celebrated.

Cancer: A Blessing or a Curse?

There is no part of our existence that is not heavily colored and dominated by the interpretation of the mind and the thoughts about what we experience. You can see this very clearly with a condition like cancer. We have all been indoctrinated to believe that cancer, when it strikes us, is a curse and that it inevitably engenders suffering. The word "cancer" fills us with fear and images of internal destruction by rapidly growing destructive masses made up of cells gone crazy. It brings up images of mutilating surgeries, poisoning by chemotherapy regimens and radiation that often contribute to killing the patient before they kill the cancer. A hundred years ago, cancer was rare, compared with today, and framed with a very different set of belief systems. It was seen more as a curiosity that rarely led to death in and of itself.

The Truth Will Set You Free

If you knew with absolute certainty what was true and what was not, would that not greatly facilitate healing from disease? If so, how can we discover and define truth? Once truth is known, can it be applied to your everyday life to help you heal? The answers to these three questions are at the foundation of our ability to heal. There are underlying absolute truths, and it is critical to be able to distinguish those from falsehoods, or untruths.

Most of what we believe is true, is not, because it stems from being indoctrinated by ego-based beliefs of others in our society and our erroneous interpretations of our own formative experiences growing up. The resultant erroneous beliefs that we hold onto with such righteousness are at the very source of our suffering and miseries.

The Science of Truth

Dr. David Hawkins, in his paradigm-changing books *Power vs. Force* and *Truth vs. Falsehood*, makes an airtight case for the fact that truth can be discerned by anyone who is truly committed and open to discovering it in literally any realm of our existence. From health care to the science arena, philosophy to politics, literature to law, and, yes, even religion—truth is definable and even measurable. Dr. Hawkins shows that just like consciousness itself, truth can be measured on a scale that is analogous to the scale of consciousness, which he was instrumental at crystallizing. The scale of consciousness is based on the premise that consciousness is identifiable and a concretely definable reality that can be calibrated. Truth as a concept correlates directly with the scale of consciousness. One can, therefore, say that truth can be calibrated using the same definitions and with the same tools that allow us to measure and calibrate consciousness. Viewing life from a state of lower consciousness is analogous to looking at a quarter from only one side and believing it is the only valid perspective. Viewing it from a higher-consciousness perspective is like looking at the same quarter and realizing that even though you can only see one side at that moment, it has another side that is temporarily out of view. One is looking at life from a narrow, limited, dualistic perspective, the other from a broader, more unlimited, unity perspective.

The Scale of Consciousness

The levels of consciousness, described in greater detail in the next chapter, correlate with our thoughts and beliefs, our emotions, our inner positionalities (how we view ourselves and others), how we process life and events, and, ultimately, even how we view our Creator; in other words, what characteristics we ascribe to the Creator (God). Each calibrated level of consciousness also defines a range of options, energy levels, possibilities, and limitations.

Ability to Heal Correlates With Level of Consciousness

Our ability to heal very much depends on where we find ourselves on the scale of consciousness. In the first chapter of this part, we talked about unresolved inner conflicts being at the very heart of illness. When you harbor an unresolved conflict, it implies that you have negative emotions as a result, which directly affects the tissues and organs of your body. Remember, disease is the brain's best solution to ensure short-term survival in the face of unresolved conflict, which threatens to overwhelm the psyche and, by extension, the brain itself.

Negative emotions, in turn, are not driven by what happens to you, but by how you interpret your experiences. This depends on your positionality; in other words, your view of yourself and others. Your positionality depends on your underlying beliefs.

It is, again, critical to note that truth cannot be discerned through the ego. The ego by definition is dualistic and exclusionary and is focused on the survival of the individual at any cost. It embodies selfishness and self-centeredness and always feels threatened. The lower levels of consciousness are dominated by the ego. Healing from physical or mental ailments by resolving the problem at its root level is nearly impossible at lower levels of awareness because of the alignment with a weak energy field defined by the lower levels of consciousness. The lower levels of consciousness are associated with disease, suffering, and life-destructive patterns, which, in turn, are linked to predominantly negative emotions, belief systems, habits, and attitudes.

Life-destructive patterns are associated with destructive physiological changes similar to those known to be synonymous with stress. These changes are associated with the sympathetic nervous system becoming overactive and include a surge in the production of adrenaline and cortisone; a decrease in the production of endorphins, serotonin, and dopamine (all "feel good" chemicals); depression of the immune system; and weakening or breakdown of organs.

This was described in the first chapter of this part; i.e., "All disease is biphasic." These are all symptoms that are part of the conflict active phase in the development of disease.

Healing Depends on Knowing and Acting on Truth

Being able to discern truth and the likelihood of acting on it is directly linked to the level of consciousness at which we are operating. Health and healing is correlated with alignment with higher consciousness, which is defined by a relatively strong energy field and is associated with life-enhancing and life-supportive patterns. Primarily positive, empowering emotions, belief systems, habits, and attitudes dominate at the higher levels of consciousness.

Life-enhancing patterns are associated with positive physiologic changes, which include a decrease in the production of adrenaline; normalization of cortisone levels; increased endorphin, serotonin, and dopamine production ("feel good" chemicals); strengthening of the immune system; and enhancement of organ functions. This correlates with the clearing of conflict-associated downloads to the brain and organs, discussed in the first chapter of this part. The energy field within and surrounding the body becomes progressively stronger as we ascend along the scale of consciousness, and at the higher levels, especially above five hundred, healing is all but assured.

At the highest levels of consciousness, miraculous, instantaneous healing is achievable at will; however, paradoxically, the importance of physical healing also diminishes because of the ultimate realization that we are not our bodies and that survival of the body is of little or no consequence. At these highest levels, it is realized that the body is just a tool that allows us to experience this particular dimension of existence and allows us to interact with others on the physical plain.

In summary, we can say that good physical and mental health is correlated with knowing and acting on truth, which generates a

positive outlook on life, a positive attitude, and happiness in general. Where you find yourself on the happiness index is maybe the best predictor of good health. If you are happy more than 50 percent of the time, you are much more likely to be healthy than if you are unhappy most of the time. If you are happy most or all of the time, good health is almost a given. Remember, your level of happiness does not depend on circumstances. Happiness is a choice.

Poor health is correlated with an inability to discern or act on truth, which leads to a generally negative outlook on life, negative attitudes, and the predominance of negative emotions, such as anger, resentment, hostility, jealousy, fear, self-pity, guilt, shame, sadness, vanity, apathy, compulsivity, and a strong tendency toward addictions.

Two Key Truths That Help Us Heal

An absolute truth that we can bank upon in our existence here on earth is that everything is interconnected. The ego sees itself as separate from everything, and everything as separate from everything else. It always acts from this perspective and is focused exclusively on survival and self-preservation at any cost. It tends to be selfish and self-centered. The higher self is able to perceive our interconnectedness with other human beings and with God's entire universe. It tends to act more selflessly and is focused on that which unites us. It always focuses on the greater good.

Another absolute truth is that there is only one moment, and that is *now*, and everything that is important is present in this moment, and everything that is not in this moment is not important. Everything outside of the present moment is an illusion. When we are obsessed with the past or the future, we are not present in our lives, and we end up experiencing the past over and over again, thinking it's the present.

Survival Programming

Also of profound importance here is that our brain contains data and programs critical to survival that are linked to the different levels of the evolutionary tree. Our beliefs, in turn, tend to be linked to these evolutionary survival programs. For example, all of us have basic animal instincts or characteristics that we have in common with all animals, including the overriding instinct to survive at any cost, which includes finding food, avoiding predators, and procreating.

The next layer of characteristics we share is with all vertebrates and includes the basic ability to learn at a rudimentary level, like how to stay away from certain repetitive threats and how to avoid falling, among other things. Animals at this level are able to perceive threats and are able to learn to avoid them.

We share common characteristics with all mammals, including giving live birth and the general tendency for mammals to take care of their young, which includes providing essential nutrients for growth through suckling. There is a greater tendency toward relationship building and a stronger group consciousness, which causes mammals to be able to share information nonverbally, or verbally, in the case of humans.

The next layer of characteristics that we share is with all primates, which have a much larger cerebrum, are much more capable of learning more intricate tasks, have the capacity for deeper relationships, and are able to feel a greater variety of emotions. At lower levels of evolution—i.e., at the level of vertebrates—emotions are rudimentary and include fear and aggression. As we go into the mammalian and progressively more so in the primate groups, we see other emotions come into play, including guilt, shame, sadness, jealousy, and anger. The next groups of characteristics that come into play are those that we share with every human being. These are characteristics shared at the level of mass consciousness with all human beings and include the tendency toward territorialism, righteousness, fear of loss, pride, and protectionism, which involves the defense of life and the protection and hoarding of resources. Also,

all human beings share basic needs, including the need for security, variety, significance, love, and intimacy.

Next, we share in common certain characteristics with a few people. For example, we congregate in groups called nations, cultures, ethnicities, and families. Each one of these groups has certain additional characteristics and feeds into the sense of the ego even more, and share the sense of significance, the desire for security, variety, and again, the desire for love and intimacy.

At the highest level, we stand alone as individuals with all the basic needs and defenses mentioned above, but also we have higher needs. We can call these the needs of the soul, which include the need to grow and learn and the need to contribute.

Almost all of our programming comes from the layers preceding the individual, which means that most of our beliefs are based on basic instincts, survival needs, and the self-interest of the individual and the group. In our world, most people still live at a lower level of consciousness, which causes them to think only of themselves (narcissistic perspective) and seldom about others, especially not about humanity as a whole or beyond that.

So, in summary, the human brain is programmed with mostly archaic programs and is programmed for survival. This is where the ego stems from and what it thrives on.

The ego is entangled with certain basic illusions that almost all human beings have in common. These illusions (false beliefs) give rise to foundational fears, which drain our energy resources available for healing. They are:

Illusion 1: The illusion of separation.

Illusion 2: The illusion that we are not enough.

Illusion 3: The illusion that we won't be loved.

Illusion 4: The illusion of suffering.

Illusion 5: The illusion of disease.

Illusion 6: The illusion of death.

The first of these illusions is the *illusion of separation*. This is the idea that we are all alone and have to protect what's ours and have to hoard as much as we can to ensure our future physical survival. This illusion of separation is the source of all the other illusions.

This illusion gives rise to the *fear that we are not enough*. Most of humanity is programmed with the notion that no matter how much we posses and no matter what we do or what achievements we make, we are never enough. Under this illusion, we always live with the belief that we are incomplete, that we are missing important characteristics, and that we are, therefore, unlovable.

The *fear that we won't be loved* in conjunction with the fear that we are not enough forms the foundation for all our other fears. Because of the illusion that we are not enough and, therefore, are unlovable, we tend to develop a fourth illusion, the illusion of suffering.

We talked earlier about the fact that *suffering* (like all the other illusions) is based on erroneous and disempowering belief systems and that we have a choice whether to see something as a curse (suffering) or as a blessing. This includes disease.

We tend to take it as a given that if we have certain symptoms and certain physical abnormalities (deviations from what's normal), we should be labeled with a *disease* . We forget that we have a choice as to whether we carry a label or not. The label itself becomes a source of conflict, depending on the type of disease we are labeled with, especially if we fear that it might culminate in our physical death.

This illusion is based on the idea that *death* of the physical body is something to fear. In fact, this is the ultimate and greatest of our fears unless we understand that even death is an illusion and that consciousness, just like energy, cannot be destroyed. This illusion, therefore, rests on a false premise; i.e., that we can go from existence to nonexistence. Consciousness, like energy, can change form and can shift in time and space, but cannot be destroyed. This is a foundational premise of quantum physics and is verified in real life by those who have had near-death experiences. Such individuals almost universally lose the fear of death after such an event, regardless of their religious affiliations or lack thereof.

We Choose Our Reality

Another important understanding to come to is that we choose our reality. Again, we referred earlier to the analogy of the roller coaster and how two people can have totally different subjective experiences, even though they experienced the same event, due to differing subjective interpretations of their experiences. They actually may experience the same or very similar emotions, but the interpretation of those emotions may be totally different. For example, both might have been terrified; in other words, they might have experienced intense fear. However, one might love the experience of being terrified while on a fast-moving roller coaster, while the other may be angry and feel overwhelmed by the same feeling of terror.

Your Thoughts Reflect Your Level of Consciousness

It is also very interesting to note that all thoughts are not created equal and that each thought has its own range of frequency. It is, therefore, clear that certain thoughts contribute to healing, and other thoughts contribute to disease. The only way to understand this effectively is to look at the scale of consciousness and to realize that research has actually been done to gauge these energy frequencies and power levels of emotions, thoughts, and belief systems. Dr. David Hawkins, in his book *Power vs. Force*, summarized this research in a way that I believe will change the way we look at this world as we know it. It has changed the way that a lot of people look at this world of ours. In his book, *Transcending the Levels of Consciousness*, he lays out a road map that anyone can follow to raise their level of consciousness and their ability to heal.

We will delve into the scale of consciousness more in the next chapter and how mass consciousness affects us. We have often heard of things like mass hysteria and have come to realize that the destructive force of one individual cannot compare to the destruc-

tive force of a group. This is born out in the history of war, where a man, Adolf Hitler, inspired a nation and was part of the evolution of a mass consciousness that led to the idea of superiority of an entire group of people.

This group fermented violence in the world as never seen before because of its belief in its own superiority over other races and ethnicities. We also see the effect of mass consciousness in disease. For example, a hundred years ago, when someone was diagnosed with cancer, the trauma of the diagnosis/prognosis would have been minimal because cancer was not really feared. It was seldom diagnosed, and it occurred seldom as a general rule. Amazingly enough, cancer was seldom fatal. People had growths on their bodies, but cancer was not thought of as a major killer. This has changed big-time in our society over the last hundred years. As we have become better and better at diagnosing cancer earlier and more and more aggressive in our battle against cancer, the war against cancer has actually made the disease worse. This seems to be the case anytime we wage war against anything. Has anybody noticed how many fruits the war on heart disease has born, or the war on diabetes, or the war on drugs, or the war on crime, the war on terrorism, and other wars? I don't mean to imply here that you just turn the other cheek, but I do believe that we can massively change outcomes and the results that we experience in this world by looking at problems not from the antagonistic perspective, but from a healing perspective. For example, when we look at cancer, as we will see in part three, "The Cure: Your Guide to Miraculous Healing," we will see that totally different outcomes can be obtained by simply seeing cancer as a state of toxicity that has migrated to a deeper level and seeing cancer as a particular biological program that has kicked in to promote the survival of the individual.

Erroneous Beliefs Tied to the Ego

Again, it's worth remembering that illusions form the basis of suffering and that illusions are tied to the ego. As a matter of fact, we can go as far as to say that the ego is bound by illusions that are based on false beliefs, with false beliefs being very heavily attached to our past experiences. The ego also is dominated by the stories about self and stories about others. Lastly, the ego is tied to the future; i.e., fears about the future and its effort to predict the future. The one thing that the ego is not bound by is the present moment or presence. Being present in your life (in the *now*) is the antithesis of ego and all of the false illusions that are related to it and bound to it.

In summary, it is critical to understand that in order to overcome suffering and to allow for healing to take place, we have to overcome illusion and shift our beliefs to encompass the idea that healing is possible. Not just possible, but inevitable. We also need to realize that true healing rarely occurs on the physical level unless it also occurs at other levels. We can temporarily influence the body with drugs, vitamins, minerals, herbs, and so on, but unless healing takes place at the higher levels—including the energy body, the emotions, the mind, and the spirit—the physical body will always revert back to a diseased state.

We also need to reframe who we are from a quantum physical perspective. Instead of the focus on the "little you," limited by a very narrow perspective and very narrow beliefs, we need to focus on the "greater you," which is far greater and more powerful than you could ever imagine and capable of miraculous healing. We also need to realize that the only place where we are empowered to be healed or to heal ourselves is in the present moment, not by focusing on the past and not by focusing on the future. Not by searching through all the stories about who you are and the stories about others. Those stories are often what limit you, especially seeing that most people's stories are very, very limited and tell about a very insignificant person with very measly prospects and huge limitations.

Four key beliefs are required for healing:

1. I want to heal.
2. I can heal.
3. I will heal.
4. I deserve to heal.

These four beliefs must be held at the deepest level of our being; otherwise, healing is not possible. There are various reasons why some have problems with one or more of these beliefs. These key beliefs will be repeated and expanded upon in some of the upcoming chapters because they are so critical in a number of different contexts that relate to healing.

I want to heal. Some have a problem with this belief because they derive a secondary gain from their illness; i.e., it gives them an excuse to avoid conflict or responsibilities that have overwhelmed them in the past.

I can heal. Some want to heal, but they fear that they cannot heal, because they believe their disease is incurable or they lack the resources to be able to heal, and so on.

I will heal. Some people want to heal, and they believe they can heal but fear they won't heal because their disease is too far advanced or they lack the will to do what they know will cure it.

I deserve to heal. This is the one that many, if not most, people have a problem with initially. They have a deep-seated belief that their disease is rightful punishment by God for their sins and that they, therefore, don't deserve to heal.

Any problems or blocks with any of these four beliefs have to be discovered and resolved in order for healing to take place. Failure to do so will lead to almost certain failure to heal, especially over the long-term.

Stress, Negative Emotions, and Your Health

Is there a link between our negative emotions and the occurrence of disease and illness? Even in conventional medicine, it is recognized that stress is a great contributor to ill health, and the link between stress and ill health runs right through negative emotions. We all know that stress and living are synonymous and that we cannot live without stress. However, again, as in the previous chapter, everything depends on your frame of mind. Looking at the roller coaster ride again as an example, it would be observed that the person who goes on the ride and experiences joy and exhilaration comes off pumped and energized and probably will want to ride a few more times before the day's out. He may even feel like he's conquered something extraordinary in his life, especially if he was fearful to start with. On the other hand, the person who experiences terror and feels overwhelmed may be quite exhausted after the ride and will certainly not want to go again, knowing that experiencing the same extreme negative emotions will lead to even more exhaustion. Again, these two people have the same experience but with totally different interpretations. We can apply the same principle to life in general and find a new, more positive framework to view the potentially stressful events associated with everyday life.

Emotions Are Gifts

All emotions are gifts that contribute to survival and self-preservation. They are like road signs in life that point us in the direction we need to go in order to heal or stay healthy if we heed them and act on them appropriately. Positive emotions tell you that you're moving in the right direction, whereas negative emotions tell you that you're moving in the wrong direction and that you may want to change your actions or your perspectives. Human beings are stubborn, though, and very often when people experience negative emotions, instead of seeing it from an empowering perspective, it becomes an excuse for compounding the problem with even more negative emotions. Instead of changing direction or mind-set, we find more reasons to feel bad. Whenever the ego gets involved with emotions, it tends to corrupt the effects of those emotions. When the ego aspect of who we are experiences a negative emotion, it contributes to the sense of separation, the sense of isolation, and the illusions that were discussed in the previous chapter.

On the other hand, when the higher self-experiences negative emotions, it looks at them as impetus for change or uses them as motivators to do what is necessary to heal what's broken. The higher self sees all potential outcomes in a positive light because it knows that even adversity leads to growth and eventual transformation.

Negative Emotions Critical to Survival

Negative emotions are critical in not just individual survival, but survival of the species. We have used negative emotions to motivate us to do things that would help our survival and the survival of our species by forcing us to take appropriate actions, depending on the threats that we face. Historically, we dealt far more with real, every-day threats that were physical in nature—for example, wild predators, human enemies, or natural disasters. We were much more likely to be attacked by an enemy that wanted to take our territory from us

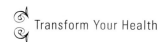

or enslave or kill us. So it was essential for survival to have negative emotions.

As we have evolved in consciousness, though, we have become more and more bound to thoughts and beliefs. Because of this, we are not so much threatened anymore by direct threats, but by the concept of a threat. What I mean by this is that we literally torture ourselves through our beliefs of what things might do to us or what might happen to us. When you look at our media, there is a constant harping on bad news and all the terrible things that happen in this world so that everybody watching has a tendency to become fearful and paranoid about a never-ending array of potential threats. Ironically, people are more concerned for their physical safety even though we are living longer than ever before and deaths through physical trauma and even from disease are at an all-time low. We also worry endlessly about disease, financial destitution, relationships, and a myriad of other threats to our health and well-being.

Emotions and Beliefs Tied Together

When you look at emotions and beliefs from an energetic perspective, there are literal differences in the range of frequencies and the energies embodied in each of these. We also should realize that the very emotions and beliefs that we hold inside of us have the potential to affect our health and our ability to heal. As a matter of fact, our emotions and beliefs overall are a direct reflection of where we find ourselves on the scale of consciousness. Dr. David Hawkins, in his history-changing research summarized in his books, including Power Vs. Force, demonstrates that each one of us operates at a specific overall level of consciousness that can be stratified and is even measurable at birth.

He also showed that the overall consciousness level continues to increase both on an individual as well as a global level, albeit very slowly. For the average individual, this growth in consciousness amounts to only a small amount during the average lifetime. In rare cases, that growth can be much larger. In his research, he

Transform Your Life

also shows that each emotion and belief can be ranked on this scale of consciousness from the least powerful progressively to the most powerful. He uses an arbitrary scale from one to a thousand. This scale denotes one as the lowest level of consciousness and one thousand as the highest level possible in concrete human form. There are only a handful of human beings in history, at least that we know of, who have reached this ultimate level of consciousness.

Every feeling or emotion that a human being can feel, every thought, belief, point of view, even actions in context can be measured and ranked on that scale. For instance, shame is at the bottom. Most people can feel or can see that when they watch somebody who is steeped in shame, there is very little energy there. You can certainly see it in their body language, the proverbial tail between the legs. When a human being is stuck at this level, the corresponding belief (the way that they look at life) is one of misery, and at this level, the emotion that is most commonly experienced is humiliation.

All emotions are *not* created equal in terms of their impact on life and our ability to heal. Each emotion has a different energy, vibrational frequency, and also a different power level. For example, guilt and shame sit at the bottom end of the scale of consciousness, meaning that anybody stuck at this level and dealing with a lot of internal guilt or shame will tend to be greatly weakened in their ability to heal. On the other end of the scale of consciousness are love, joy, and peace. When someone is at peace within their self is filled with joy (that is not situational, but a premise upon which they live and thrive) and loves their self and others unconditionally, their ability to heal is markedly greater. So from shame at the bottom to guilt, grief, fear, anger, and pride higher up (but still in the negative range of emotions), we see this limitation in regards to healing. The closer we get to the level of courage, which is beyond pride, the stronger the level of emotional energy becomes.

Our ability to heal is directly correlated with the emotions that we carry and directly correlated with the overall level of consciousness at which we operate. At the lower levels of consciousness, healing is almost impossible, and even if it occurs, it is temporary and

rapidly reversed. On the other hand, at the higher end of the scale of consciousness, healing is not just easier to accomplish, but also inevitable in some ways. For instance, when a human being, a group, or a nation as a whole is stuck at the level of shame or guilt, there is a dramatic and tremendous impairment in the individual's ability to heal and the nation as a whole.

Another example is someone at the level of guilt who tends to take on blame very easily and tends to blame others (the victim mentality). Their approach to life is that of being self-destructive and destructive to others. What is interesting is even the way they look at life and God is defined by their overarching level of consciousness. At the lower levels of consciousness, there is also a total failure to be able to comprehend that bad luck or victimhood or failure in general is premised on faulty perception of reality, and not on true reality itself.

For instance, at the level of guilt, life perspective is one of evil lurking around every corner and that one forever has to be fearful of evil. God is characterized primarily by being a vindictive creator out to get you if you don't comply. As we go up on the scale of consciousness through apathy, which is associated with hopelessness, grief, tragedy, and regret, next we get to the level of fear. The actual level of energy at the level of fear is increased when compared with that of shame, guilt, and apathy. This can be observed when you watch somebody in fear or somebody wracked with anxiety. The person is certainly more animated, with more energy running through his body than in those experiencing lower-level emotions. At the level of fear, life is frightening, and there are lots and lots of things to be frightened about. Anxiety predominates at that level, and there's a tendency to withdraw from that by which we feel threatened.

At that level of consciousness, God is likely to be viewed as a punitive God that is out to punish, but always for good reason because you are a sinner, because you're bad. Once we go beyond fear, we get to the level of desire, which is the level of addiction, enslavement, and craving. Life is viewed as disappointing, and God is seen as a denying God that denies us happiness because of our

weaknesses, because of all of our addictions, because of a lack of commitment, and so on. At these lower levels of consciousness, true healing is nearly impossible to achieve and unlikely to last.

At the next level of anger, the predominating emotion that people harbor is that of hate. Aggression is used frequently here as a way to deal with others and others are seen as antagonists. God is seen as vengeful and out to punish harshly when we are noncompliant with his laws or requirements. The next level is the level of pride, which is also the level of vanity and self-conceit. At the level of vanity, healing is unlikely to occur, because the person's focus is on appearances and status. There tends to be an obsessive focus on possessions, having more things and better things than others. Individuals at this level also tend to have a hard time with aging, especially with the physical changes that accompany it.

In these lower domains, from shame up to pride, healing is very hard to achieve even though symptoms can still be managed at these levels. People in this realm of consciousness tend to look for the quick fix, tend to look for instant gratification and instant relief from symptoms. They are far more likely to be the ones paying very little attention to their habits and the possible underlying root causes of their health challenges and far more likely to be self-destructive, either because they are simply unconscious to what is happening to them or willfully ignorant by literally thumbing their noses at what they know is true about lifestyles and what they are doing to themselves through self-destructive habits and patterns. There is also an overall tendency here to blame others for what ails us or even to blame God, and an overall resistance to take responsibility for our failings and challenges.

At the lower levels of consciousness, we are strongly bound to the ego and its tendency to selfishness and self-centeredness. The ego always sees itself as separate from everything and is focused on its own survival at any cost. It cannot conceive of the concept that disease is a solution and a blessing, not a curse. At the higher levels of consciousness, this concept is progressively easier to understand and to act upon.

Positive Emotions Heal

At higher levels of consciousness, above two hundred on Dr. Hawkins' scale of consciousness, true healing becomes progressively more achievable the higher we ascend. At this level, we are able to make a critical leap from nonintegrity to integrity and from being a victim and at the mercy of others to taking progressively more control of our universe, especially our inner universe. The ego is transcended progressively more and more, and we are able to perceive the universe in progressively more nonlinear terms. The ego can only perceive of the universe as linear and, therefore, cannot perceive of a quantum physical, nonlinear universe where anything is possible. By ascending to higher realms of consciousness, it becomes progressively easier to conceive of quantum physics, the fact that we live in a nonlinear universe where quantum leaps are possible and can conceive of and even experience miraculous healing.

At the first level of consciousness above the line denoting positive and negative levels of consciousness, we move into the realm of *courage*, which is associated with affirmation. In other words, this reflects the first step that is critical to take toward healing. At this level, people are more likely to use affirmations to affirm positive habits, to affirm their health or the ability to heal, and will tend to be more empowered to make better choices and to take positive steps toward their own healing. The life you live at this level is one where true healing becomes feasible. God at this level and above starts being seen as a constructive versus a destructive creative force. At the level of courage, we perceive of a Creator that allows or permits us to heal.

The next step is the level of *neutrality*, at which we start giving up the need to judge ourselves and others. We start transcending the need to judge everything from a dualistic perspective as good or bad, positive or negative, black or white, right or wrong, and so forth. We are able to discern that which is constructive from that which is destructive without limiting ourselves to strictly dualistic thinking patterns. This is also the level where we learn to be able

to trust, where we start being able to trust ourselves and others to act with integrity. We move toward a more positive view of life and tend to take on more constructive, health-promoting habits in order to experience more optimal health. Our focus tends to be on more positive thoughts, and daily stress becomes progressively easier to transcend. This is also the level of release; i.e., being able to release what holds us back and what sabotages us in our lives. The perspective at this level of life is that we are satisfied, that where we are and what we are achieving is satisfactory. We see a God that is enabling and enables us to succeed in life.

The next level is the level of *willingness*. For healing, this is a very important level to achieve, because here we become willing to change, to move out of our comfort zones, and to take on the challenge of transforming our habits. People at this level are hard workers and enthusiastic learners who have a great capacity and desire to learn from others. This is the level that we have to attain to become predominantly optimistic in our pursuit of health and healing and to transcend pessimism. This is also the level where we start creating through positive intent and start using intention as a creative force. We become more goal-oriented rather than just letting chaos reign. In order to heal, we first must be able to visualize and see ourselves achieving that goal. At this level, we start becoming filled with hope and start seeing God as an inspirational force willing us toward greater achievements in our lives, including the healing of what ails us. Hope is a very powerful entity when it comes to healing, but unfortunately in itself is still relatively weak because hoping to get better is not the same as knowing that we can get better.

The level of *acceptance* is signified by the emotion of forgiveness and transcendence. In order to resolve negative emotions and to gain much greater traction in our healing efforts, we have to learn that forgiveness is the key to happiness. An unforgiving heart hurts no one but oneself. At the level of acceptance, it also becomes possible to transcend our limitations. At this level, healing can take place rapidly, sometimes so rapidly that it appears semi-miraculous because we are able to transcend severe self-destructive habits that

have heretofore been harder to overcome. This is the level where self-discipline and mastery become more prominent and where long-term goals become much more important than short-term goals. At this level, life also becomes harmonious and God is seen as a merciful God, not out to punish us for our transgressions. At this level, we realize that we punish ourselves through our ignorance and self-destructive perspectives and actions.

Next is the level of *reason*, which is the level of understanding, the level of scientific achievement, and the level of abstraction. At this level, life becomes far more meaningful. We start being able to gain an objective understanding of the intricacies of our universe, how things work and interrelate. Healing at this level of consciousness becomes more easily achievable because we are able to figure out from a rational perspective why we are ill. We are able to gain a much deeper understanding of what lies at the root of illness. A more rational, systematic approach to healing is now possible. We can now also gain more clarity on the links between emotions, buried feelings, belief systems, and the roles they all play in illness and regaining health. Our view of life at this level is that life makes sense and we see our Creator as a God of wisdom that bestows upon us the capacity to gain wisdom and perceive truth even though our capacity to understand subjective truth is still limited.

This level also represents a glass ceiling that most of humanity never transcends. Oftentimes, understanding becomes a limitation because there are certain things that simply cannot be understood through the intellect; for instance, intuition and unconditional love.

The next level of consciousness is the level of *love* which represents the level where we are able to start seeing the big picture, to discern essence, and to see the greater good. Intuition becomes a major tool for discernment, which holds huge implications in healing. At this level, it is far easier to see and resolve the conflicts that underlie all illness and misery in general. This is the level of revelation, where we become capable of insights so powerful and profound that they have the ability to heal almost instantly. The premise at this level is to always endeavor to see the whole, to take a nondual-

istic perspective, to have reverence for all of God's creation. This is the level of true happiness. God is seen as an unconditionally loving Creator, and we start to perceive of God as being in everything, and that everything and everyone has a divine essence.

The level of *joy* is characterized by a state of joyful being, which comes from within. The joy felt at this level reflects the overall state of being and has nothing to do with outer circumstances. In fact, infinite patience and perseverance even in the face of prolonged adversity and deep compassion for all living beings is characteristic of those who have evolved to this level. Everything and everyone, including self, is seen as beautiful and complete, and a divine presence is perceived and felt within oneself and in our surrounding universe. We see ourselves as one with our Creator. This is also the level at which unconditional love becomes pervasive and constant regardless of circumstances, and everything is seen as a miracle. Serenity abounds. Healing at this level becomes almost effortless, and being in the mere presence of someone at this level often acts as a catalyst for miraculous shifts in belief and thought, which, in turn, allows healing to take place, sometimes so rapidly that we call it miraculous.

At the levels beyond this, a point is reached where the physical body itself matters very little and the concept of disease holds no sway. Yet paradoxically, healing can take place instantly if desired or useful. For instance, so that one can maintain a presence in physical form in order to contribute to the transformation in consciousness of mankind. At these highest levels of consciousness, what happens to the physical vehicle is neither here nor there. The concept of death of the physical vehicle holds no more energy. These are the levels beyond thought where infinite peace and silence replace thinking almost entirely. At the highest level of consciousness, the term "enlightenment" is used. At this level, we have returned to pure consciousness.

In summary, our bodies are manifestations in the visible universe of our invisible universe of beliefs, thoughts, feelings, and emotions. Our very cells, including our DNA, hold within them the

memory of perfect health, which can be unleashed when we uncover and release unresolved inner conflicts and their accompanying buried feelings and emotions. Spontaneous healing of every disease known to mankind has been recorded through the ages. There is no such thing as an incurable disease. In almost all cases of spontaneous healing recorded in literature, there was a shift in consciousness that preceded the spontaneous healing. Whether it is the release of unforgiveness, letting go of guilt, fear, or rage, or the embrace of courage, willingness to change, or learning to love ourselves unconditionally, there is always a major shift in perception and release of negative emotions that take place.

As in so many cases of spontaneous, miraculous healing, so too does each one of us have the capacity to heal any disease that we are confronted with if we have the willingness and capacity to shift our perception and our consciousness. Our feelings and emotions are our guides and are reflected in the body itself as symptoms and diseases. Our emotions are also, in turn, reflections of our prevailing thought patterns and by extension our beliefs. In order to heal, it is necessary to discover and heal negative emotions and their accompanying unresolved conflicts. Each symptom and every disease are direct reflections of very specific negative emotions and very specific unresolved conflicts that program for them.

Relationships and Your Health

Dysfunctional, codependent, adversarial relationships contribute to illness and suffering. Healing from disease, therefore, requires the healing of our relationships.

Like our overall health, our emotions, and our belief systems, our relationships are also a reflection of our inner universe and define our capacity to heal. When we look at most of humanity, we see very few instances where relationships truly transcend the ego and the lower attractor fields of negative emotions and negative beliefs. More and more people are experiencing glimpses of transcendence in their relationships, but find it very hard to stay on a consistent spiritual track.

Relationships as Your Mirror

Relationships are in many ways the ultimate mirror for us to evaluate what our underlying wounds are and our underlying beliefs are about life and about our universe. If the mirror that we're looking into is filled with misery, frustration, anger, resentment, and other negative emotions, we tend to blame those that we are in relationship with for those emotions. This is one of the main reasons why the divorce rate continues to skyrocket in this country and why in many countries, people don't even get married anymore. Seems like the whole marriage paradigm is fracturing at its very foundations, and families are splitting apart and fragmenting all across the globe. Most of our grandparents and great-grandparents grew up in an era

when families were close-knit, when parents seldom got divorced and stayed together through thick and thin, sickness and health, till death do us part. Children honored their parents even if the parents were cruel and sometimes misguided in the way they raised their kids. Extended families were pretty much the norm, where the children and grandchildren in families would settle in the same town or same district as the rest of the family and where family get-togethers were held on a regular basis.

This paradigm has certainly changed dramatically with most families split apart, either through divorce or simply through the pursuit of the American dream and the dream of material abundance or independence. People move sometimes across the globe in pursuit of their occupational dreams, often at great emotional cost to their families.

Our relationships with others around us can be compared to school, where our toughest, but most important, teachers are those who are closest to us. Most of us experience our greatest negative emotions related to our very closest relationships, like those with our spouses, our children, our parents, extended family, closest friends, and business associates. As a matter of fact, as a general rule, the closer you are to somebody, the more sensitive you are to the person's negative emotions and criticisms. When you don't have a deep relationship with somebody, generally, it would probably bother you less if you are criticized by them or have negative emotions projected at you.

The Quality of Your Relationships Reflects Your Level of Consciousness

The quality of our relationships and the type of people we are surrounded with correlate in general with our overall level of consciousness and are often the most obvious observable reflection of where we find ourselves on this scale. Our level of consciousness acts as an attractor field, drawing to us those people and experiences that are congruent with that overall level. This means, for example, that

if you are surrounded by angry, resentful people who are projecting these emotions at you, you are in all likelihood operating at the corresponding level of consciousness. On the other hand, if you are surrounded with kind, compassionate, loving human beings who project these positive emotions at you, you are likely operating at the corresponding higher level of consciousness. This is called the law of attraction.

It is important to note that we are referring to our overall level of consciousness. Most human beings experience emotions that span the full spectrum of both positive and negative emotions at times. Most have days or moments when we seem to be surrounded by negativity and everything seems to go wrong, and good days, when we seem to be surrounded by angels and everything seems to go right.

When we look at humanity as a whole, the majority of humankind finds themselves at a level of consciousness below the level of integrity, truth telling, and constructiveness in general (level of two hundred). These are the levels just below the level of courage, which is the level where relationships become more generally constructive rather than destructive. The relationships that we have with others, in a general sense, reflect where we find ourselves on the scale of consciousness. It makes sense that interpersonal conflicts will be rather ubiquitous for those operating at the lower end of the scale of consciousness.

As we ascend to higher consciousness levels, there is generally a progressive decrease in the frequency and intensity of interpersonal conflicts. At the higher levels—i.e., above the level of love—interpersonal conflicts are rare and of low intensity, and by the time we get to the level of peace and above, there is almost complete cessation of interpersonal conflicts.

The Purpose of Relationships

It is interesting to note that the purpose of relationships shifts, depending on where you find yourself on the scale of consciousness.

At the lower end of the scale of consciousness, the purpose of relationships revolves around the fulfillment of four basic survival needs at almost any cost, even if fulfillment of these needs has negative implications or consequences. These needs include first, the need for security, stability, and consistency; second, the need for variety, stimulation, and excitement; third, the need for significance and status; and fourth, the need for love, intimacy, and affection.

First is the need for security, stability, and consistency. Most people who get married or get involved in a committed relationship think that their main motivation is having fallen in love. More often than not, they discover that the warm and fuzzy feelings experienced early in the relationship give way to rude awakenings. The reason is that what is initially interpreted as love stemmed from the hidden need for security and belonging, a sense of stability. They tend to try and replace their parents with another human being that reminds them in some way of their parents and can take their place as a pillar of strength in their lives.

The next basic purpose of relationships is the need for variety, stimulation, and excitement. Oftentimes, these first two needs, the need for security and the need for variety, are at odds with each other. On the one hand, we want stability, so we want a relationship that will always stay the same. We want the person we are married to or living with and wake up next to every day, to be the same person day after day. We like consistency and predictability and feel very insecure when that person changes. Men often blame women for this when they go through PMS, the woman that you thought you were married to for the first twenty-one days of her cycle suddenly changes in the last seven days, and you don't quite know who you are married to anymore. All the stability and consistency can get boring, however, so we also have a basic need for stimulus; in other words, for excitement and variety. When we're married to the same person for a long time, we start getting bored, and we start craving change of some kind. We want the person with us to transform him or herself in some way to meet our need for variety and stimulation; otherwise, we often go searching for variety and stimulation

in someone or something else. This is a key reason for the epidemic of infidelity in our society. And if you can't find variety in another person, you go find stimulation or excitement via some other means, like alcohol, drugs, or food.

The third purpose of relationships is to meet the need for significance and status. This is also a basic ego-based need that all of us have when operating at lower levels of consciousness. We want to be seen as significant and important by others. A large part of our pursuit of wealth, education, even marriage is focused on meeting this particular need. We want to keep up with the Joneses or outdo them if we can. We want the high-status job, the big paycheck, the nice house and cars, and the good-looking husband or wife. We pursue the elusive perfect figure and perfect weight, and get surgery to "upgrade" our appearance so that we can feel significant in the eyes of friends and family and society as a whole.

The fourth purpose of relationships is to meet the need for love, intimacy, and affection. This need is so important that it imperils our very physical existence when we do not receive or are unable to express love and affection for extended periods of time, regardless of age. We are social animals from the moment we are born till the moment we die, so isolation in a social sense equates to death. It is one of the main reasons why people do so poorly in the average nursing home, especially once they become less mobile. Nursing home staff members often feel reluctant to connect with their patrons. They don't want to get too close because that would entail suffering on their part if the patients die, which they routinely do in a setting like this. We see the same problem in orphanages around the world, where children are often not given a lot of love and affection for similar reasons of not wanting to get too close because of the pain it entails to see little ones suffer.

In Romania, for example, during the early stages of the AIDS epidemic when it was thought that AIDS was communicable through direct human contact and not just through sexual contact or needles, literally thousands of AIDS orphans died in orphanages, where they were treated at arm's length by the staff, who were afraid

to pick them up because of what turned out to be a baseless fear that they could contract AIDS from these children, and also because they did not want to connect with these children who they thought were going to die and feel the pain of losing them. As it was later discovered, many of them were not even infected with the AIDS virus even though their parents had AIDS. This basic human need is also a need that is critically linked with health. In our society, because of the high levels of relationship dysfunction, loss of love and affection is all too common. In the absence of this critical human need being met, disease and death are far more likely.

The purpose of relationships at the higher levels of consciousness changes dramatically and become more spiritual in nature. Even at higher levels of consciousness, there is a desire for our basic human needs to be fulfilled, but we tend to meet even these basic needs in constructive, healthy and uplifting ways. There are at least two additional human needs that come into play and that we have a strong urge to meet in higher-level relationships. They include first, the need to grow; and second, the need to contribute.

1. The need to grow. Our closest relationships represent those relationships that we tend to learn the most from when we are committed to growth rather than being victims. The more antagonistic our relationships, the more it reflects that we are operating at a lower level of consciousness and are operating strictly from the ego. Most of us grow only when we have to, through intense pain and suffering, whether it is as a result of dysfunctional relationships or illness. Both have the effect of pushing us out of our comfort zones and in a state of pain and discomfort. We are far more likely to take active steps to break out of the misery than if we are comfortable with everything as it is. In order to end suffering or to minimize the suffering that we need to go through in order to grow, we have to focus on wanting to grow instead of always waiting for life to make

us so miserable that we have no choice but to grow or risk annihilation.

2. The need to contribute (altruism). At the higher levels of consciousness, we also become more conscious of the need to contribute. As we will see later, contributing to others is a critical part of healing. In order to be healed, we have to take on the responsibility of being healers. Each one of us is a healer, not just those with twelve years of training and with diplomas on their walls. Each one of us becomes a healer when we have committed ourselves to our own healing. Even the very level of consciousness at which we operate has a constructive or diminishing effect on those that we are in relationship with or even humanity as a whole. In Dr. David Hawkins' book Power vs. Force and in his other books, this point is demonstrated repeatedly, the reason being that positive emotions, thoughts, and beliefs are logarithmically far more powerful than negative emotions, thoughts, and beliefs. Dr. Hawkins makes the point that a few loving thoughts, for example, counter and neutralize the negative impact of thousands of negative thoughts. In the same way, you find that the power embodied by one human being functioning at the higher end of the scale of consciousness—i.e., at the level of unconditional love—counters the negative energetic impact of thousands of people operating at the lower end of the scale.

When our singular motive in life becomes to grow and to be of service to others, it has a major transformative effect on us, our relationships, our ability to heal, and even on the health and well-being of strangers that we are surrounded by. That impact reaches across time and space and impacts not just a few individuals close to us, but humanity as a whole. One such man is Jesus, who even now, more

than two thousand years since His birth, continues to have a huge positive impact on this world.

Relationships at the Source of Unresolved Conflicts

We discussed in the chapter titled "Unresolved Inner Conflicts and the Root Causes of Illness" that at the root of illness are unresolved conflicts that are downloaded to a small focus in the brain and/or the body when such a conflict threatens the integrity of the brain as a whole. Unresolved conflicts, in turn, stem from our erroneous beliefs and the resultant negative thoughts and emotions that accompany them. In the final analysis, unresolved conflicts result from the fact that we are unconscious or operating at lower levels of consciousness linked to a greater tendency to hold erroneous beliefs, feel negative emotions, and think negative thoughts. This is most clearly reflected in our relationships.

You could say that the vast majority of our unresolved conflicts stem from and are reflected in how we relate to each other and to the universe around us in general and even to our Creator. Our relationships, therefore, are at the source of most of illness.

Disease-causing Conflicts That Stem from Relationships

Relational conflicts such as the *conflicts of separation* and the *conflicts of territory*, program for diseases in tissues and organs related to the ectoderm, which includes the brain cortex, the outer layer of the skin, the inner layer of the coronary arteries, the mucous membranes of the bladder, the cervix, the nose, the esophagus, the ureter (connects the bladder to the kidney) parts of the rectum, parts of the kidneys, nails, hair follicles, and so on.

Relational conflicts such as *conflicts of self-devaluation* program for diseases in the tissues and organs related to the new brain, medul-

lar layer, which includes bones, muscles, and connective tissues, such as ligaments and tendons.

Relational conflicts such as *conflicts of protection*—those related to being attacked, the threat of attack, the threat of losing the integrity of the body or symbolic loss of integrity—and *conflicts of the nest* (home), nurturing, or feeding of others program for disease in the tissues and organs related to the old brain, cerebellum, which include the cerebellum itself, parts of the breasts, deeper layer of the skin (dermis), outer (protective) layer of the lungs, inner abdominal cavity, heart, and brain.

In diseases related to the brain stem and the tissues and organs related to it, which include vital organs, such as the liver, large parts of the kidneys, intestinal tract, lungs, sex organs, heart muscle, and hormone-producing glands, the conflicts are vital in nature. *Vital conflicts* would include *morsel conflicts*, which relate to the intake of or excretion of food (or fecal) morsels or something symbolic for food or fecal matter. It also could relate to *water-based conflicts* (i.e., too much or too little); *air supply conflicts* (i.e., not enough air); and *pro-creation conflicts* (i.e., with the loss of a child or what the brain reads as symbolic of these conflicts). All these disease-producing conflicts are related to real or symbolic threats to our physical existence and usually relate to other human beings and can come from within our group or from outside our group.

As mentioned before, relationships are like school. In order to transform your health, you have to transform your relationships and the unresolved conflicts that are at the root of not just your health problems, but your relationship challenges, too. The quality of your relationships also reflects where you are in consciousness and can act as a major impetus for personal growth, which, in turn, greatly facilitates healing.

Spiritual Roots of Illness

We are sick because we do not know who we are and because of our belief that we are separate from our Creator, and therefore separate from each other. This is the source of all suffering.

We discussed earlier that illness occurs as a direct result of unresolved conflicts and that unresolved conflicts are related to our false beliefs, negative thoughts and emotions, and our dysfunctional relationships with each other as human beings. Among all the false beliefs that we embrace that contribute to illness there is one that is foundational to all others: the belief that we are separate from our Source, our Creator, and, therefore, separate from each other. This belief also forms the foundation of the egocentric mind-set.

Where we reside on the scale of consciousness directly relates to how we see ourselves in relationship to our Source; i.e., our Creator. It also directly relates to our ability to heal and our ability to help others to heal. In order to be able to heal, we need to learn to distinguish between fulfilling our spiritual needs and simple religiosity. Fulfilling our spiritual needs is critical to achieving health, whereas simple religiosity sometimes runs counter to our ability to heal. What most people forget is that we are all products of our domestication. Most of our beliefs are inherited or programmed into us during childhood. What we were taught by our parents, our siblings, other family members, friends, our schools, and religious institutions forms the bulk of our belief systems. It is only when we start operating at a higher level of consciousness that we are able to discern: (1) between empowering and disempowering beliefs and

become able to choose accordingly, and (2) which of our beliefs are based on truth, which are based on partial truth, and which are based on untruth, or falsehood.

Religion

Where you find yourself on the globe at birth pretty much defines your basic religious beliefs. For example, if you're born in a country like the United States, you're far more likely to grow up in a Christian household holding Christian beliefs, whereas somebody born in a country like Iraq is far more likely to grow up in a Muslim household holding Muslim beliefs. If you happen to be born in Tibet, it would be very unusual for you not to grow up as a Buddhist, and so forth. More people in this world have been killed in the name of religion than in the name of any other cause, and what is frightening is that the numbers killed in the name of religion continue to mount as we enter deeper into the twenty-first century. Man has taken the arrogance of his religious beliefs to unbelievable levels and, because of his righteousness regarding his beliefs and thoughts, tries to force those upon others, contributing not just to illness on a personal level but also to the sickness of our societies in general.

There is a saying that goes as follows: "You can either be right or you can be happy but not both [at the same time]." Comedian Ralphie May stated this quip as a reference to married men who want to stay married, but I believe it is a powerful principle to live by in relationships in general. By definition when you insist that you are right, you are making someone else wrong, and when someone else insists that they are right and you are wrong, unhappiness inevitably follows. This is maybe the single biggest reason for human misery, including wars, domestic violence, the epidemic of divorces in our society, and tension between people of different races, ethnicities, and religions. This statement has nothing to do with truth or falsehood. Claiming that you are right and someone else is wrong is an ego construct; whereas, our ability to discern truth is defined by the level of consciousness that we are operating at. At the higher levels

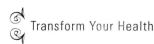

of consciousness, we gradually transcend the ego and therefore transcend the need to be right or for that matter the need to prove that we are right. Truth cannot prove itself. Truth can only be discerned. The moment you claim truth and feel compelled to fight for truth, you lose your grasp on it because the very act of having to fight for it means that you don't have it or that you have lost track of it. Truth cannot be proven. It can only be lived and embodied.

Fearing Evil and Fearing Hell

Does our belief in hell make any sense? The truth is that we needn't fear hell or fear going to hell after we die because a large percentage of humanity frame their existence as hellish; in other words, they feel like they are in hell while they're alive. It should be reassuring to recognize that based on the characteristics used to describe evil, evil resides at the weaker end of the scale of consciousness. The emotions and beliefs characteristic of the higher end of the scale of consciousness, such as unconditional love, joy, and peace, are logarithmically much more powerful than the emotions and beliefs characteristic of evil, such as vindictiveness, condemnation, disdainfulness, destructiveness, abdication, elimination, and despondency.

Another common fear is that evil may be hard to recognize and, therefore, make us more vulnerable to its potential to claim us as its victim. Again, this is an erroneous belief that stems from the ego, which cannot discern truth from untruth. The higher self, which is synonymous with our divine essence and which by definition does not fall sway to the ego and its false beliefs, is easily able to discern truth from untruth. The higher self is intuitive by nature and can easily discern ego-based beliefs and those individuals who countenance them from divinely inspired beliefs and those among us who are committed to the higher path of integrity, which leads us back toward divinity. For all these reasons, evil need not be feared. Fear and being judgmental are negative emotions and characteristics that have to be resolved in order for healing to take place. This includes the fear of evil and religious-based judgment.

Transform Your Life

How You See Yourself Is Synonymous With How You See God

It is no small irony that there is a strong congruency between how people see themselves and their own lives and how they see their Creator in terms of overall characteristics, or the other way around. If they see their Creator as a punitive, disdainful, condemning, vindictive, or despising God, chances are that is how they feel about and act toward others and themselves. Healing in this environment is very unlikely to occur. On the other hand, if they see God as an unconditionally loving, wise, merciful, and inspiring presence, chances are they feel that way about their fellow man and act accordingly. Healing in this kind of environment is far more likely to occur. How people see themselves and their Creator also helps define the attractor field that they project into the universe that draws to them the experiences and people that are congruent with what they put out in thought and belief.

I have reminded some of my patients who are most afraid to shift their belief systems that the vast majority of mothers in this world would never even be able to imagine, let alone do to their children what people think God will do to His children who happen to believe wrong or happen to have been born in the wrong place—things like sending them to hell for all eternity because they chose the wrong religion.

When ascribing characteristics to our Creator, it is also important to note the following truths. You cannot feel judgment and forgiveness at the same time. You cannot feel connected and choose isolation at the same time. You cannot feel love and harbor hatred or anger or even look down upon other souls at the same time. You cannot feel joy and sadness at the same time. Peace is not possible when you hold onto the fear of the unknown or the fear that you somehow will be tainted if you harbor a thought of unity instead of a thought of separation, even as part of your religious beliefs.

God Is Omnipresent, Omniscient, and Omnipotent

One God and Father of all, who is above all, and through all, and in you all.

Ephesians 4:6

For of Him, and through Him, and to Him, are all things: to whom be glory for ever. Amen

Romans 11:36

"Can any hide himself in secret places that I shall not see him?" saith the LORD. "Do not I fill heaven and earth?" saith the LORD.

Jeremiah 23:24

The real dilemma and the deepest underlying root of all disease and misery is the belief that we are separate; i.e., that we have a duality-based mind-set versus a unity-based mind-set. The Bible makes it clear in so many ways and in so many places that God is omnipresent, omniscient, and omnipotent. All the world's great religions agree on this one basic principle. Therefore, the essence of the divine is within all of us, no matter how many evil deeds we have committed or how many evil thoughts we have had. God loves all of us, even the fallen angel, even Hitler or other modern-day evildoers. What is expressed as evil is analogous to disease in the body. It stems from unresolved conflicts and wounds inflicted through our genealogy and through our parents via our "project purpose" or during childhood. If we realize this, we might also choose to look at criminality, unethical behavior, cruelty, and so forth in a slightly different light. It does not mean we make excuses for it or turn a blind eye to it or fail to protect ourselves and our loved ones from it. It just means being more compassionate and less arrogant in our judgment and condemnation of others.

Adversity Leads to Personal and Societal Growth

It is good to remember that even those great evildoers, such as Hitler, were the instigators for massive growth in consciousness. Hitler, by antagonizing the forces of complacency and narcissism so prevalent at that time in the world, helped to deepen the consciousness of our society. Certainly, this was not his conscious motive, but the end result of this antagonism led to a massive shift in consciousness. The 9/11 attacks here in America did the same thing in many ways. Even though those who perpetrated those dastardly deeds were evil their very deeds helped to bring people in this country and around the world together, and those deeds also triggered a deepening of consciousness. Each time calamity strikes, we as human beings deepen spiritually at some level, and we get to choose again and again whether to unite or to be separate. If we choose separation, we choose more misery and disease. We cannot on the one hand want to heal and on the other hand hold on to the thought that we are somehow separate from others. That doesn't make sense. In other words, when you yearn for healing of yourself, you can only have it when you also want it for others.

You don't have to wait for the rest of mankind to gain consciousness before you can heal. You can alleviate your own suffering by making the shift in consciousness anytime you choose, and your suffering will lessen or resolve. This happens simply because we all have the power to be able to reframe suffering. Healing spiritual wounds is so important that overall healing cannot take place unless we reframe our spiritual beliefs to the point where we no longer exclude or condemn others. A condemning heart cannot heal. I've found that some patients will make steady progress toward healing, but will fall just short of full recovery and will start getting sick again. When I start investigating, I often find that at least part of the problem is an unresolved conflict related to their religious belief systems. This conflict makes it impossible for them to let go of the fear of being condemned by God if they stop condemning others for

their religious beliefs; however, they don't realize that by condemning others they condemn themselves. The truth is that we live in a nonlinear universe where we cannot escape the reality that what we inflict upon others, we ultimately inflict upon ourselves in a karmic sense. That includes judgment and condemnation, which lead to deep-seated guilt and, ultimately, to a conflict deserving health. (A conflict deserving health means I feel deep down that I don't deserve to be healthy; in other words, I am conflicted about whether or not I deserve to be healthy.) From a karmic perspective, our judgment and condemnation also ensure that we will draw to us the judgment and condemnation of others in order to allow the soul to learn through that experience.

In order to heal, we have to give up our religious-based judgments, including condemnation of others who do not share our beliefs and guilt regarding our past-perceived violations of our own religious beliefs. We have to give up religious-based fear of God's condemnation and fear of evil and of hell. Holding on to fear is not conducive to healing. As long as you are condemning others, no matter how strong you feel about your belief systems and no matter how great your convictions are about the rightness of your beliefs, if your belief system is dualistic in nature and is based on the idea of separation from others and from God, you will not be able to heal fully and completely. The bottom line is that complete healing is not possible when you carry any unresolved conflicts.

> Judge not, that ye be not judged. For with what judgment ye judge, ye shall be judged: and with what measure ye mete, it shall be measured to you again.
>
> Mathew 7:1–2

> And if any man hear my words, and believe not, I judge him not: for I came not to judge the world, but to save the world.
>
> John 12:47

Part III

The Cure

Your Guide to Miraculous Healing

A Shift in Consciousness

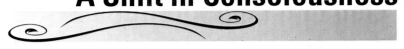

This is the third part of the book, and it is focused on solutions to promote self-healing. A shift in consciousness is an essential part of healing. Most of us have heard of or know individuals who have experienced miracles in their health. These are individuals who were told that they had an irreversible or incurable disease and somehow, in spite of these diagnoses or pronunciations by their health care providers, got better. In those cases, where we have detailed histories of exactly what occurred, it is very telling that every single one of these individuals described a marked shift in his or her consciousness or in his or her state of consciousness.

Dr. David Hawkins, in his history-changing book *Power vs. Force*, makes the unequivocal observation that there is a direct association between the calibrated level of energy (consciousness) and the capacity for healing. Individuals at the lower end of the scale of consciousness find it nearly impossible to heal, and the best they can do is attempt to treat symptoms when they occur. Healing at a deeper level is not possible in most of these situations. On the other hand, those at the higher levels of consciousness not only have a higher level of awareness, but also an easier time in terms of their ability to heal, and are often healers themselves in some capacity.

As a matter of fact, everyone is a potential healer. Healing is not just for those who have studied for years and have gone through formal education to become healers. Everyone has the capacity to help others heal and to be conduits for healing. A mother is a healer to her children through her love and caring. A teacher is a healer for

her students through the love and care that she brings to her profession. The janitor is a healer of the environment for children to learn in even though he may work behind the scenes and get very little recognition. His spirit of caring and how he takes care of the premises that he cleans affects the energy in that location either positively or negatively.

All the great healers of history and of today are individuals who find themselves at the higher end of the scale of consciousness. Individuals at high levels of consciousness seem to radiate healing energy, and just being around them often brings about profound changes in those in their company. This is especially true if an individual in the company of a healer shares an intention to be healed and the healer acts as a conduit for healing. In other words, what is happening is through the power of intention; higher spiritual energy lowers and reverses disease-based energy. It is important to remember here what most of us learn through our religious beliefs, not just in Christianity, but in other religions as well. The belief that we were created in God's image and likeness helps us to understand that our birthright is to be healthy and vibrant and it is not a given that we have to suffer with disease and illness as we go through life. Dr. Wayne W. Dyer describes it most succinctly when he says that in order to heal we have to reconnect to the disease-free, loving, perfection from which we came.

When we discussed the roots of illness, we discussed the importance of our thoughts, emotions, and also our behaviors in the formation of disease in our bodies. What is really happening is that negative thoughts, emotions, and behaviors create resistance to the flow of energy in our bodies and cloud consciousness. Healing, therefore, requires unclouded consciousness and removal of all blocks to energy flow, including this critical area of thoughts, emotions, and behaviors. We can go further and say that our emotions follow our thoughts, and our behaviors follow our emotions.

It is mentioned over and over in most books on health how important lifestyle is. What often is forgotten, though, is that lifestyle involves action that follows beliefs, thoughts, and emotions. In

order to become motivated to live a healthy lifestyle and to be able to intuit what is healthy for us as individuals, we have to change our thoughts and emotions, which start with a shift in our beliefs. Another key is to discover our hidden negative intentions (subconscious intentions) and replace them with empowering intentions for healing.

In further examining this area, let's review the three hidden intentions that are important to know about that often sabotage our ability to heal. I would say that probably 60 percent to 70 percent of people have one or more of these key blocks present, as a result making it impossible for them to heal.

1. Conflict regarding a desire for health.
2. Conflict regarding a belief that wellness is possible.
3. Conflict deserving health.

When most patients come to a physician like me, who practices holistic medicine, they truly do want to get healthy and want to be healthy. However, when I was still practicing conventional medicine, it was quite common for me to see patients who had a hidden agenda or a vested interest in their disease, whether they were consciously aware of it or not. When we study the realm of unresolved inner conflicts as it relates to health, we come to realize that a lot of illness results from a subconscious conflict that makes illness the better option between two bad potential outcomes. For example, if you have a hard time saying no and a hard time defining your boundaries, and you have anger or resentment toward a loved one, you have a choice to withdraw from the person, actively risking wrath of that individual or becoming sick with an illness that protects you against their aggression or an invasion of your privacy. An example of this would be fibromyalgia syndrome, which is signified by physical pain of a musculoskeletal nature associated with insomnia, chronic fatigue, and often depression.

The second obstacle to healing: There are many people who want to get healthy, but have a deep-seated belief that they are beyond the

point of being able to heal. This usually results from indoctrination by the medical community, by friends and family, or by the media that a disease is incurable and even that the disease might have a high likelihood of being too severe, leading to debility or even death. When you are caught up in such a belief system, no matter how much you want to heal, the likelihood of this is minuscule until you have dramatically shifted that belief system toward a strong abiding belief that you can be healed.

Most individuals who have open-mindedness about the options for treatment of their illness are being treated in a more holistic setting by, for example, a holistic health care provider and will tend to stay strong on the belief that they can be healed or that they can be healthy again.

The third obstacle to healing is very common and very hard to diagnose. The reason is that most people are not even aware that they have this subconscious obstacle to healing. This conflict regarding health is linked to a deep-seated subconscious belief that somehow the disease that they're struggling with is just punishment for bad behavior or for being "sinners" in God's eyes. In a society where religion plays an important part, where a lot of religions still feed on guilt complexes, this is even easier to understand. As we become more mature in our spiritual or religious beliefs and we start identifying so-called bad behavior with ego-mindedness and so-called good behavior with divine consciousness or the essence of who we are, it becomes a lot easier to let go of these feelings of guilt and to take on a greater ability to heal.

Healing Through Recall

Recall healing: "To heal from any illness, it is necessary and sufficient to remove the source of conflict within oneself."

—Claude Sabbah

That sounds easy enough, doesn't it? The first problem, of course, is first to become aware of our unresolved inner conflicts. The second problem is how to resolve or clear the conflict in order to allow the body to heal.

Becoming aware: "Everything that comes back to awareness does not come back as a destiny."

—Karl Jung

Why Are Most People Unaware of Their Disease-triggering Conflicts?

By definition, when an inner conflict arises that is too great for the conscious mind to bear, it downloads to the brain and to the body as illness, clearing it from the conscious mind. Therefore, it becomes hard to access directly through our waking consciousness. This is called a mini-maxi schizophrenia, which means we develop a blind spot and can't see or are not aware of our own conflicts. This is a critical biological adaptation inherent to this phenomenon. This adaptation enhances the chances of short-term survival by clear-

Transform Your Life

ing the conflict from waking consciousness, which would otherwise remain the focus of consciousness at that moment, which in terms of our biology would be potentially catastrophic. Short-term survival in nature depends in large part on constant awareness to avoid ever-present dangers to survival. Take, for example, a primitive human being, at the mercy of nature, the elements, and dangerous predators, just to mention a few. If that human becomes consumed with an inner conflict at any point in time, his awareness would lapse and more than likely put him in mortal danger. On the other hand, when the unresolved conflict downloads to a smaller part of the brain and to the body, it releases waking consciousness instantly to focus on avoiding or overcoming more imminent threats to survival.

Unfortunately, there is a price to pay for this extraordinary biological adaptation. Even though the likelihood of short-term survival is enhanced, if the conflict is intense enough, it may program for an acute illness even if it resolves quickly. If the conflict remains unresolved—in other words, remains downloaded—the consequences may include a chronic disease linked to the specific conflict. Eventually, the chronic illness likely will impair the quality of life and may threaten long-term survival.

The Solution Is Recalling the Conflict and Resolving or Reframing It

Fortunately, there are ways to gain access to the underlying disease-causing conflicts. However, because unresolved conflicts are usually hidden from waking consciousness, we may initially need the assistance of someone schooled in Recall Healing to help us figure out the underlying unresolved conflict that is behind our symptoms or illnesses. We also may want to learn more about Recall Healing in general so that we can figure out what the most common conflicts are that are linked to our particular symptoms or illnesses.

First, attempt to recall the conflicts that occurred just before you started to have symptoms. Draw a timeline that has the exact

point in time when you started having a particular symptom, if you can remember. This may help to jog your memory regarding what was happening in your life shortly before the onset of the particular symptom. In the case of more serious illnesses, you may want to think back up to two years prior and even up to ten years in rare cases in order to find the triggering conflict. Also, make the effort to discover the programming conflict by going back all the way starting from one year of age to just before the triggering conflict occurred. In the case of very traumatic experiences, the programming and triggering conflict may be one and the same event.

Discovering the programming and triggering conflicts that activate the biological pathways to disease formation is critical here. You do this by asking questions that will help you build awareness of your disease or symptom timelines. The following questions might be helpful: When did I start having symptoms of illness?

What happened that was either psychologically or physically traumatic before the symptoms of illness arose that might have become a triggering conflict? What happened earlier in life, years or even decades before the symptoms started, that was traumatic in some way and that could have become a programming conflict?

Second, use your body as a guide, specifically, by knowing the biological meaning of symptoms and diseases in terms of the underlying conflicts that are typically linked to them. The body and the personal characteristics of an individual can be read like a textbook: Each symptom and each pathological condition, each emotional state, personality trait, fear, habit, and choice we make tells a story about our underlying psychological conflicts, our programming and conditioning, and our genealogy.

Here is where conventional medicine can play a helpful role. Well-trained practitioners in natural or alternative medicine also can be of great assistance here. Knowing your diagnosis can be very helpful in tracking down the underlying conflict.

Each disease or symptom can be associated with one or more conflict. Pairing your specific history of emotional or physical trau-

mas with the potential conflicts that can program for your condition can make conflict tracking a lot easier.

Third, discovering the psychological conflicts of your parents before, during, and after your conception and birth will help you discover what is called your "project purpose." The psychological conflicts of the parents during the period spanning from nine months before conception to one year after birth become the biological conflict of the child, with biological pathways for disease formation set that early on. This is another survival tool and is essential for the parents to be able to function at a level in this world where they have the greatest chance at being able to support their offspring and continue to procreate.

For example, if a woman falls pregnant in order to "keep her man" because of stress in the relationship, the child conceived will carry the conflict of "keeping mommy and daddy together." Later on in life, if there is discord between the mother and the father, or if they get divorced, the child's subconscious conflict will escalate to the degree where they may become physically ill with an illness representative of the conflict of separation, like eczema.

Fourth, discover the genealogical downloads that are linked to the background or history of your family (birth family and/or adoptive family), especially as it relates to unresolved conflicts in the family that tend to get passed from generation to generation. These conflicts are carried epigenetically. In other words, they are carried on your genes, not in your genes. They can make a major contribution to disease formation, especially those diseases that are familial (that run in the family). It has been established that we get major biological conflict downloads from as far back as four generations and possibly more. Helpful information here includes birth order; family secrets; unexpected, traumatic losses suffered in the family; and so on.

The most critical part of healing is becoming fully aware of our unresolved inner programming and triggering conflicts. Awareness is responsible for 60 percent to 80 percent of healing. Just like a

shadow resolves in the light, the conflict will resolve when the light of consciousness is shed upon it.

We can resolve conflicts in one of three ways:

1. We can find solutions to the conflict, e.g., heal a broken relationship through counseling or remove ourselves or someone else from a conflict situation, such as a woman abused by her spouse or threatened with physical harm.

2. We can reframe the conflict so that it becomes neutral in our consciousness; i.e., by total and unconditional forgiveness of someone who has hurt us in some way.

3. Transcend a conflict through love, compassion, insight, awareness, finding a spiritual framework, or positive action.

Other tools can be used, like reflection, meditation, prayer, emotional freedom technique, psychological counseling, hypnosis, neurolinguistic programming, timeline therapy, or family constellation therapy.

It is also essential to increase mental and physical energy through healthy nutrition, exercise, supplementation of essential nutrients, enough rest, sunlight, fresh air, avoidance of environmental and food-based toxins, and enough water intake.

Three additional invaluable steps include:

1. Opening up to a deeper connection with the eternal, creative force in our universe (God), which is only accessible within each of us and not outside of us. The answers to our health problems are within each of us ready to be accessed when we are ready and willing to open up to divine wisdom.

2. Also, foster an attitude of gratitude for everything, including your illnesses. They are part of the magical survival system within you that gives you the greatest

opportunities to continue on your path in this physical world of ours.

3. As you heal, realize that you, too, are a healer. When you heal your wounds, you change the consciousness in your family and in the world and assist in the healing of others. Love is the healing force within each of us that empowers us to heal and to help others to heal.

Knowledge frees us, and love heals.

—Anonymous

A Synopsis of Some of Our Most Common Health Challenges

The following section is not meant to cover every system or every illness that can possibly afflict a human being, and it is not intended to be a comprehensive review of the illnesses that will be discussed. It is strictly meant to give some context to what has already been discussed in the first chapter of part two, and the first part of this chapter. Most of it is in an abbreviated format to facilitate rapid review of these examples.

Cardiovascular Diseases

Myocardial infarction [heart attack/coronary thrombosis] is still the most common cause of death in the industrialized world. The primary conflict programming for this disease involves a conflict related to the loss of territory (either real or symbolic). A good example is the story of Kenneth Lay, the founder and CEO of the energy giant ENRON.

Mr. Lay was CEO of ENRON when the company was in its prime, and when it became one of the richest companies in America, almost overnight. He was indicted for major felonies, such as fraud, when ENRON went down in flames in the early part of this

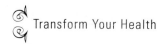

decade and was blamed by the media, politicians, and investors all over America for mismanagement. Mr. Lay had to await trial for well over a year while all of this was going down, becoming more and more an object of scorn, when finally his case went to trial, and he was found guilty on a number of charges and sentenced to jail. Within six weeks of his sentencing, he had a massive heart attack, from which he was unable to recover. As a matter of fact, he died almost instantly.

Another great example is an experiment that shows how a conflict involving loss of territory is induced in a dog, leading to a fatal heart attack in the animal.

One particular investigator did an experiment with a dog (dog A) that was brought to a farm with a spacious meadow adjacent to the farmhouse and was given free rein to roam and explore the entire property at will and was kept well-fed on flavorful dog food, including fresh meat. He was allowed to experience this freedom and abundance for an extended period of time. Then one day, they built a small dog pen overlooking the meadow, placed the dog in the dog pen, and started feeding him strictly dry dog food and water.

The same day, another dog (dog B) was brought to the farm and unleashed onto the property, giving this dog the same opportunity to roam freely. It was given the same flavorful dog food and meat daily as the other dog had previously been given. All dog A could do was watch from his dog pen as this other dog took over his territory. For the first few days, dog A barked incessantly when he saw dog B running across the meadow as he had done. This went on for about nine months, during which dog A also was given plenty of food and water, but kept penned up. After exactly nine months, dog B was taken away from the farm, and dog A was released from his dog pen to once again roam free. The dog was obviously ecstatic as he ran around, enjoying his freedom again, but within forty-eight hours, he had a massive heart attack and died on the spot. This example demonstrates that other living creatures can be affected just like humans by deep-felt stress leading to conflicts becoming biological and programming for disease.

During the *conflict active phase* (which means the conflict is still present and ongoing), the coronary arteries must increase their diameter for greater blood flow needed in order for one to fight for his territory. The most rapid and economical way is for the enlargement of the inner diameter through ulceration of the endothelial layer and the relaxation of smooth muscle.

During the *repair phase* (which means the conflict has been resolved), everything is reversed and blood vessel diameter is decreased rapidly by the healing of ulceration and the contraction of smooth muscle in the coronary arteries. This phase is characterized by the inflammation of the inner lining of the blood vessel and the activation of clotting pathways. If the conflict is of short duration and of mild or moderate intensity, symptoms will be mild, including slight chest pain (mild angina). If the conflict is of longer duration, lasting nine months or more, and is of very high intensity, it will almost always result in a fatal heart attack, unless drastic action is taken to modify this repair phase; i.e., high-dose aspirin, nitroglycerin, clot-busting drugs, or steroids. Cardiac bypass surgery, balloon catheterizations, or stent also may be life-saving during this period.

Hypertension involves a masculine-type biological conflict related to defending or protecting or gaining territory. This may include feeling pressured to be more successful or to have to work harder, do more, solve more problems in order to please others or oneself. There is usually great difficulty putting things aside at night, with the brain continuing to work on "problems" during sleep. It also can relate to a love lock; i.e., when one feels "shut out" by a loved one, such as a spouse, and when one feels that one has to "win" that love back. Another conflict that can result in the development of hypertension involves a conflict related to liquids or fear for survival affecting the kidneys and causing the kidneys to hold back fluid.

Congestive Heart Failure (CHF) involves a biological conflict related to the loss of territory with a feeling of powerlessness. It also can relate to feeling powerless in a key relationship; e.g., relationship with spouse, with children, with parents. It also can relate to

the conflict of self-depreciation related to the competence of one's physical heart.

Digestive Tract Diseases

The main biological conflicts affecting the system involve morsel conflicts, which means the conflict relates to things that we cannot digest, assimilate, or get rid of. Each organ has subtle tonalities and subtonalities.

All conflicts can be real, imaginary, symbolic, or virtual. Here are some examples using the gastro intestinal tract (GI tract) to demonstrate how this applies.

1.   Real: When something real is swallowed and is indigestible, it leads to an obstruction or causes injury to the esophagus, stomach, or lower down in the intestinal tract, i.e. like a sharp piece of bone. This can lead to a stomach or esophageal cancer.
2.   Imaginary: This means it is not based on reality but on imagination. Our imagination is so powerful that effects on the body can be every bit as powerful as a real indigestible object. This relates to the felt experience; in other words, "conflict feels like an indigestible object stuck in my gut."
3.   Symbolic: This may involve, for example, words from someone such as "I cannot digest" or that "sticks in my craw.
4.   Virtual conflicts: This means it only exists in imagination, not in reality. It could happen, or it could exist, e.g., a massive hurricane hitting New York City, which could devastate the city, but has extremely low odds of happening.

It is important to remember that the biological conflicts that program for any illness involving any organ system can fall into any of these four categories listed above.

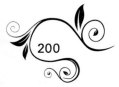

Transform Your Life

The biological conflicts for ear, nose, and throat conditions relate to the statement, "I cannot catch the morsel" An example might be a child needing to hear the words "I love you" spoken by the mother. The words are symbolic of a morsel of food or nutrition, and the child wants to "grab" those loving worlds from the mother's mouth when the child feels in conflict with the mother.

Tonsillitis is an example of a condition affecting this part of the body. The biological conflict of this condition is related to the inability to swallow something, either real or symbolic, i.e. harsh words of condemnation spoken to a child by a parent figure or having to choke back words. During the conflict active phase the tonsils enlarge, whereas inflammation (tonsillitis) or a tonsil abscess occurs during the healing phase with the breakdown of the enlarged tonsils with an organism like a streptococcal bacteria involved in this break down process. With this condition, find out what words were "choked back" in the twenty-four-hour period prior to the development of sore throat.

The biological conflict for the esophagus relates to the statements, "I cannot swallow that," such as someone's antagonism or resistance, or "I thought I had something or grabbed something, but it got taken away." For example, someone thought he had a certain job but as soon as he started he got laid off.

The biological conflict for the stomach involves something that you cannot digest, usually related to an annoyance or recent conflict within my family clan; for example, ongoing antagonism between a husband and wife, with the husband not being able to digest insults thrown at him on a regular basis.

The biological conflict for the small intestine involves something you can't assimilate; in other words, "I cannot absorb it or accept it" or my being wants to "flush it"; i.e., overbearing and controlling behavior of a parent toward a teenager.

The biological conflict of the colon (including the ascending, transverse, descending, and sigmoid colon) involves something vile or unpleasant that you cannot "eliminate" or that is of a long-standing nature. In other words, there is something symbolic for fecal

matter that cannot be cleared; this may include resentment, anger, or sadness.

The biological conflict for the rectum involves something you can't forgive, that you're stuck with, that you hold on to, or that cannot be overcome. A couple of examples would be deep resentment toward a business partner who acted unethically causing the business to collapse or the loss of a dearly beloved family member that you just can not let go of.

Diarrhea is an example of a condition affecting the upper intestinal tract (small bowel and/or stomach). The biological conflict of this condition can involve any of the following elements.

- It can be related to something that "I am unable to digest or assimilate" with or without an element of powerlessness.
- It can be something disgusting that you are letting go of in order to move forward.
- It can be something that triggers a visceral fear, for example when someone gets the runs due to stage fright before they go on stage.
- It can be related to actual food that has gone bad or has gotten contaminated. However, even if the explanation is an infectious agent or poisoned food, you will always also find a biological conflict that matches the disease, as you tend to find in any accident and the actual injury sustained during the accident.

Constipation is an example of a condition affecting the lower intestinal tract, mainly the colon. The biological conflict can involve any of the following elements.

- It can be related to conflict of active separation, such as holding onto someone who is either threatening to pull away or has already left or has died.
- It can be a conflict related to fear of not being able

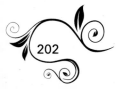

to "move something all the way through." This can be related to the "project purpose;" for example, the mother's fear or preoccupation with a baby's bowel movements or the baby not eating enough or not being able to digest properly.

- It can involve a conflict related to the inability to move the lower body. This also relates to the reality that inactivity or paralysis contributes greatly to the development of constipation.
- It can involve a conflict of identity in one's territory; i.e., feeling like one does not belong in the home or work environment leads to numbness of the rectum and signals failure to defecate.
- It can involve a conflict of something that you cannot forgive or that you hold on to.

Diseases of the upper GI tract tend to be related to more recent morsel conflicts, and those more distant in time or even ancient—for example genealogical wounds or project purpose wounds—tend to affect the lower digestive tract.

Metabolic Diseases

Obesity or problems with excess weight or excess fat tissue may involve one or more of several biological conflicts listed below.

I. Conflict of abandonment: This is possibly the most powerful conflict programming for obesity. In nature, abandonment by the mother means starvation and death. We identify food with mother and motherly love. Therefore, even if the mother does not abandon the child physically, but just symbolically, it becomes a program for obesity. This symbolic abandonment may include failure to breast-feed or failure to do so long enough. For example, a mother breast-feeds a baby until she is three months old and is a stay-at-

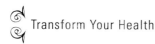

home mom for those three months, doting on her baby every moment, and then suddenly returns to work when the baby is three months old. She immediately stops breast-feeding, switches the baby to formula, and puts her in day care with a dozen other babies who are competing for attention from two or three caretakers. This baby will experience a conflict of abandonment. If a baby experiences abandonment, he will biologically begin storing a portion of what he ingests as fat. Fat provides nine calories per gram, while sugars and protein provide only four calories per gram. The body, therefore, has a biological incentive to store fat.

When we gain weight, biologically, we are easier to spot, and it increases the chances of rejoining the flock and overcoming abandonment. It also has safety implications: "For when I am bigger, I am more imposing and less likely to be attacked by smaller predators."

2. Conflict of aesthetics: Devaluation is the conflict that tends to be the one that locks in obesity and the condition of being overweight. As soon as a child is big enough to gain a sense of self and begins comparing the self to others, the child gains a perception of being fat. In the United States, that perception may not even be valid, but it creates a conflict, regardless. In one study, twelve-year-old girls were surveyed on how they saw themselves. Over 70 percent perceived themselves as overweight or fat, even though only 15 percent met the criteria. Over 50 percent of those girls had already been on a diet at least once in an attempt to lose weight. The conflict related to "my figure" often also is associated with a biological conflict of needing to be bigger. "I am too little and in danger of abandonment or threat from the outside. When I become more imposing, I will no longer be in danger, and my mother will notice me more easily." This locks the obesity in

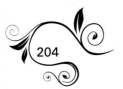

place so that even when the conscious mind wants to lose weight, the subconscious conflict persists.

The conflict around your figure must be resolved before an attempt is made to lose weight. It is a mistake to wait until you lose weight to resolve the conflict of aesthetic devaluation. This conflict also is referred to as the conflict of the mirror. One of the reasons that it is so hard to clear is because of the thousands of daily reminders that we are fat, from our image in the mirror to the oversized clothes that we put on to the difficulty moving around to the way others look at us, and so on.

3. Conflict regarding an indigestible lack: This is almost universal among humans in industrialized countries, such as the United States. Our human species has a built in biological code related to nurturing by the mother. A baby must be nurtured by the mother for the first three years of life. The young child must remain by his mother until he is at least six years old. However, at this age, the child becomes too heavy and is better able to outrun a predator by his own power than in his mother's arms. Whatever the infant is fed when it is weaned prematurely from its mother's breast becomes their fixation later in life. This fixation increases if additional stress or conflict is added through emotional trauma or high stress in the family. For example, the child may take on the fear of the parent of not enough food to feed the family, possibly due to financial hardships.

4. Conflict related to needing to protect myself against danger: This is a conflict related to a threat to one's survival, which can be countered by increasing in size. Why do we store in the form of fat instead of in the form of muscle or bone? Because fat is more voluminous and lighter mass. It provides more energy for a potential conflict that may threaten its survival. For

instance, a child who is molested or an adult who is raped will store fat in order to be more imposing and to be able to survive.

5. Conflict of identity: This is related to a conflict regarding the right to exist, to express oneself, to offer opinions, or to have one's own territory.

6. Conflict of anger and resentment toward others: This is related to those feeling attacked by the system (in the family, in society, or at school). By being larger, they are less likely to get attacked and will distance themselves from aggression and pressure that is directed at them. For example, a woman gains weight during a challenging marriage and during divorce, or a woman gains weight after being raped (especially in the buttock-pelvic girdle). She becomes fatter to protect herself and make herself of less attraction to such behaviors.

7. Conflict regarding helping others/carrying the burdens of others: This is often seen in the more empathetic members of our health care profession and even in some of the great leaders in history.

8. Conflict related to resistance: An example of this might be someone who is fed up with a spouse or fed up with the family or the system. Through weight gain, the periphery is pushed back or held at a distance.

9. Conflict related to loss: And example of this might be a mother who loses a baby who weighed ten pounds and dies at birth. She may almost instantly gain ten pounds or maintain a ten-pound weight gain to compensate for the loss of her child.

Diabetes or hyperglycemia in general relates to a masculine-type conflict which involves resistance or having to "fight" or be ready to fight. My body prepares by increasing available sugar levels in the blood stream. More specifically, in diabetes, there is a very high-level

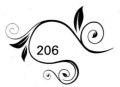

and longstanding conflict of resistance with an element of disgust ("repugnance"). For instance, you have to resist something or someone who also disgusts you.

The conflict programming for hypoglycemia is in some ways the exact opposite of hyperglycemia. In other words it tends to be a feminine-type conflict that relates to avoiding the fight. Yet in some ways the conflict is similar to hyperglycemia because there is an element of resistance with an overwhelming fear or disgust ("repugnance"). For example, a little girl is molested by the grandfather whom she looks up to but is scared of. One day he asks her to kiss him, to stick her tongue in his mouth. This overwhelms her with disgust, even though she complies because of the fear of disappointing him or the fear of rejection.

There is a minor component of resistance even though she gives in. This becomes the programming conflict of hypoglycemic attacks in the future any time she feels "disgusted with something that she resists."

The primary biological conflict of *chronic fatigue syndrome* has to do with a conflict of direction or to lose one's way. In other words it might manifest if you get lost or feel separated from one's flock—family, friends, social, or religious groups.

Chronic fatigue relates to the conjunction of five different conflicts related to the same situation or event.

1. Conflict of direction (adrenal glands—cortical area).
2. Conflict of self-devaluation.
3. Conflict of powerlessness (myopathy).
4. Conflict of displacement (oblique/from the side or to the side).
5. Conflict related to stress of survival or related to liquids (kidneys).

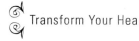
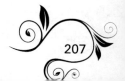

Olfactory System Diseases

The biological conflict of the *common cold* relates to something that smells foul in my territory, for example, something stinks, and you want it out of your territory, or something bad is going on behind your back. Another example is the "snorting bull" that literally wants to "blow" an invader or uninvited guest away from its territory. Rhinitis, or the common cold, usually also involves a conflict of separation related to something that smells foul. The common cold usually occurs during the healing phase of a slight general human conflict related to territory and involves inflammation of the nasal mucous membranes. During the conflict phase, there is ulceration of the nasal mucous membrane which typically is asymptomatic followed by the healing phase during which the symptoms of the cold appear.

The biological conflict of the *flu* also involves a general human conflict related to territory (GHCRT), and the symptoms of the flu occur during the repair phase or healing phase of this conflict. Influenza relates to a brief, but very intense, conflict in the family or kinship circle or in the work environment (extended family.) Again, this relates to a general human conflict related to territory. For example a relationship for a period of time becomes "unbearable," with a sudden aversion to one who is normally loved and cherished. Again the symptoms of influenza occur during the healing phase, with the flu virus present to accelerate healing of the ulceration of the mucous membranes of the throat, the nose, and the bronchial tubes.

Respiratory System Diseases

The biological conflict of *sinusitis* is a fear or apprehension in connection with "smell" or something that smells foul. An example would be an intruder in your personal space (conflict of territory). It is related to a mild to moderate general human conflict related to territory. The symptoms of sinusitis happen during the healing or repair phase after the resolution of the conflict, whereas ulceration of the sinus mucous membranes occur during the conflict active phase. The biological conflict associated with *bronchitis* is a

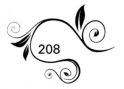

conflict related to threat in one's territory, but the enemy has not yet invaded, though it's imminent, for example, a threat related to work, to family, to marriage, or to children. This is a general human conflict regarding a "menace in my territory" (GHCMT). It may also involve arguments with or criticism by coworkers, spouses, children, or other family members. If the element of fear dominates, the left bronchial tube tends to be affected, whereas if the element of conflict is more related to one's territory, the right bronchial tube tends to be affected. The bronchial mucous membranes ulcerate during the conflict phase and swell up and start healing during the healing phase with the additional element of infectious organisms, which may be viral or bacterial. If the conflict is less severe and of shorter duration, it can program for bronchitis or the flu.

The biological conflict associated with *bronchial cancer* is similar to that of bronchitis (a GHCMT), except it tends to be of longer duration and of high intensity. This conflict is usually experienced in a climate of oppression and being in a position of weakness or of being dominated.

The biological conflict associated with *asthma* is often linked with the concept of suffocation or feeling smothered. For example, "I feel like my parents are smothering me with their high expectations or they are not giving me my space." Another common example is "I feel like I have to be perfect but yet a part of me wants to rebel." Another common conflict associated with asthma has to do with not wanting to be where you are or wanting to be in two places at the same time. A common example would be a child of divorced parents that wants to be with both parents at the same time but can't or wants to be living with the parent who does not have custody. Asthma can also be linked to the fear of actual death through suffocation or being smothered and not being able to breathe freely. The conflict plays out in the physical body by enlarging the diameter of the bronchial tubes by reducing muscle mass or by ulcerating mucous membrane. During the healing phase, muscle and mucous membrane initially swell, reducing the diameter of the bronchial tubes, but they eventually return to normal after the repair phase.

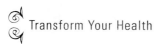

An asthmatic attack often occurs or reaches its peak during the epileptoid phase. The intensity of the attack is related to the intensity of the conflict (see page 138) and the duration of the conflict.

The biological conflict associated with *pneumonia* typically is a conflict related to an intense fear of death or of suffocation. This fear can be related to oneself or toward a loved one or more than one loved one.

The biological conflict of *adenocarcinoma of the lungs*, or lung cancer, is the same as for pneumonia, but of higher intensity and longer duration. A common situation where this occurs is when another cancer or life threatening health problem is diagnosed and very negative words are spoken about that illness leading to a very intense fear of death. This is the type of conflict which programs for metastatic cancer in the lungs. When fear is about another possibly dying, a solitary lesion usually is the result. When the fear is of oneself dying, multiple lesions are the result. Pneumonia always occurs during the healing phase or repair phase of the conflict, whereas adenocarcinoma of the lungs always occurs during the conflict active phase. There are usually relatively few, if any, symptoms present during the conflict active phase unless the tumor becomes big enough to impair airflow into the lungs causing shortness of breath. This is one reason why this type of cancer is typically diagnosed very late in its development.

The biological conflict for *tuberculosis* is similar to that of alveolar lung cancer. The TB occurs during the healing phase of a cancer of the pulmonary alveoli after the resolution of an intense or longstanding fear of death; i.e., during wartime for those living in a war zone.

Urinary Tract System Diseases

Bladder infection (cystitis) is a rather common urinary tract system complaint. The biological conflict of bladder infections is the inability to mark one's territory, to determine one's position, to find one's bearings, or to organize one's territory. It may also relate to a loss of one's organizational plan.

Breast Diseases

Breast cancer is the second most common type of cancer among women and continues to escalate in incidence. The biological conflict associated with the most common type of breast cancers is a conflict of the nest that is of high intensity and of long duration. In a right-handed woman, the left breast relates to conflict of the nest associated with mothering. It is typically a drama related to someone you are mothering; i.e., your children, your animal, your house, your pet project, enterprise, grandparent, or cherished husband that is sick. In a right-handed woman, the right breast will tend to be related to a conflict of the nest that is nonmothering in nature or what is called an "extended" nest conflict. Here it is typically a drama involving someone you are caring for but not mothering—a sibling, friend, parent, grandparent, or partner. In a left-handed woman, things are reversed, and a conflict of the nest associated with mothering will affect the right breast, whereas a conflict of the nest that is nonmothering in nature will affect the left breast.

Thyroid Diseases

There are many different thyroid diseases—too many to list here. Diseases of the thyroid are usually associated with conflicts relating to time and fear associated with it, leading to either a tendency to accelerate or decelerate.

Hypothyroidism (underproduction of thyroid hormones) develops when there is a sense of being overwhelmed and an inability to move fast enough. For example, you might feel like your hands are tied, like you are devalued and powerless, or you may have too much to accomplish and not enough time to accomplish it. The conflict leads to a need to decelerate, to slow down in order to handle the overwhelming circumstances. The thyroid gland obliges and acts in a biologically congruent manner by reducing thyroid hormone production.

With *hyperthyroidism* (overproduction of thyroid hormones), the conflict is of a similar nature, but the difference is that the feel-

ing of being overwhelmed comes with a feeling that everything can be accomplished if only I can accelerate, if I spend more and more hours working or if I work as fast as I can.

Autoimmune thyroid disease is a common cause for hypothyroidism. The biological conflict relates to feeling cornered or completely overwhelmed with a component of feeling complete powerlessness.

Bone Diseases

The biological conflict that programs for *osteoporosis* revolves around a generalized long-standing conflict of devaluation. Bone thinning takes place during the conflict active phase. So as long as someone is suffering from a profound generalized conflict of devaluation, there will be a generalized progressive decrease in bone mass. In a country like the U.S. there is a lot more devaluation linked with aging and being "past our prime." For example, when a woman in America has dedicated her life to raising children and running the household and has foregone a career in order to fill this role, there is a tendency toward feeling deeply devalued when the children grow up, leave home, don't need Mom as much any more, and don't stay in contact as regularly. Pair that with financial dependence on a spouse that may not show as much appreciation for the contribution made to the household by the dedicated wife and mother. This picture is very different in countries like China and Japan where the elderly are respected, treated well, honored, and shown more appreciation. Osteoporosis rates in these two countries are a fraction of that which we see in America, even though there tends to be much lower calcium consumption, dairy consumption, and female hormone replacement therapy in those countries compared to America.

The biological conflict of *osteoarthritis* relates to a more specific conflict of devaluation which has unique characteristics depending on which joint is involved, in other words the specific tonality of the devaluation conflict is related to the area or joint that is involved.

Transform Your Life

Rheumatological Diseases

The autoimmunity indicates a notion of self-destruction. Arthritis and arthritic conditions are related to conflicts of devaluation or depreciation. Rheumatological diseases manifest during the healing phase, but with repeated reactivation of the conflict phase followed by healing phases the arthritic condition becomes chronic and progressive.

During the conflict phase, there is destruction of cartilage without pain; inflammation and pain occur during the healing phase. In rheumatoid arthritis the conflict of depreciation which programs for the disease is linked to certain specific movements or gestures associated through the felt experience with devaluation.

The dominant *shoulder*, in other words the right shoulder in a right handed person or visa versa in a left handed person is linked to devaluation related to my own identity, in other words how I see myself. The opposite or "non dominant" shoulder is linked to a biological conflict related to self-devaluation in relationship to another family member or family as a whole.

The biological conflict of the *elbow* involves a depreciation linked to performance of one's job or work. The dominant elbow is affected when a conflict occurs related to having to perform work or a task that we don't feel like doing, whereas with the nondominant elbow, the conflict relates to having to do a job that you feel you cannot manage because you feel incompetent or overwhelmed.

The biological conflict of the *wrist* has to do with self-devaluation related to my ability to perform a specific manual task or related to having to be the intermediary between conflicting parties and feeling incapable of success in that role.

The biological conflict of the *fingers* is related to execution of or action related to work, such as in writing, grasping, holding, pulling, or squeezing.

The biological conflict of the *ribs* involves depreciation in relationship with family members; for instance, not feeling loved enough. The four upper ribs relate to members who are older, such as a parent or a grandparent. The four middle ribs relate to those

who are the same or similar age, such as a sibling or a cousin. The four lower ribs relate to those who are descendants; i.e., children and grandchildren.

The biological conflict of the *spinal column* and the vertebrae in general revolve around conflicts of depreciation. Each vertebrae and each region of the vertebral column involve a specific subtonality of a conflict of devaluation. For example the cervical vertebrae (C1 through C7) relate to either intellectual depreciation (C1, C2), depreciation related to loss of morale or loss of inner peace because of disagreement in the family (C3, 4, 5), or depreciation related to injustice in the family or in the workplace (C6, 7, T1).

Lyme Disease

The biological conflict of Lyme disease is related to separation from clan. The incidence of Lyme disease is rapidly rising in the United States because of the fragmentation of the core family structure in our society. It relates to the pursuit of wealth and status, leading to the separation by distance from loved ones.

Liver Disease

The liver originates from the endodermic embryonic layer and therefore is linked to the brainstem and conflicts revolving around immediate survival. The main conflict of the liver has to do with lack or deprivation related to food, such as an intestinal illness that threatens to cause starvation by blocking the intestinal tract (for example, colon cancer) or lack of something symbolic of food or sustenance, including money, family, or faith.

Pancreatic Disease

The biological conflict of the pancreas is similar to that of the rest of the intestinal tract which has to do with morsel conflicts; e.g., you were forced to swallow something either real or symbolic, but you resent it deeply. It can also be a conflict involving deep disgrace,

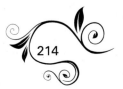

Transform Your Life

something that is indigestible or most terrible to digest, or conflict of fear related to inheritance, as in the case of ignominy. An example may be: "My father does not recognize me, or I do not carry the name of my father." You then think you are therefore not eligible to receive your share of his inheritance, again either real or symbolic.

Crohn's Disease

The inflammation of the bowel, which is a key symptom of Crohn's disease, occurs during the repair phase or healing phase of its biological conflict. It relates to a morsel conflict—something sordid and indigestible associated with the fear of lack of something vital often associated with family clan, something that cannot be assimilated within the family.

Leukemia

The biological conflict of leukemia is a major deep seated, global, and long-standing conflict of devaluation usually related to ones family or blood line. The disease occurs during the repair phase of the conflict, which causes the bone marrow to go from a suppression of white blood cell production during the conflict active phase to a massive overproduction during the repair phase of the conflict.

Lymphoma

The biological conflict of lymphoma also relates to self-devaluation, but of a lower degree than that of leukemia, and occurs in relationship to the part of the skeleton or organ corresponding to the conflict. The mild devaluation often also is associated with a conflict of fear and the feeling of being unable to protect or defend oneself or the inability to eliminate something. The lymphoma always occurs during the healing phase of the conflict.

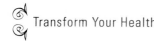

Prostate Cancer

The biological conflict relates to feeling of impotence as a man. For example, you may feel unable to protect your children or grandchildren or feel you cannot please your partner anymore. It also can be a conflict related to feeling impotent in relationship to money or business. For example perhaps you cannot make enough money to satisfy your family or to take proper care of your family.

Cervical Cancer

The biological conflict of cervical cancer has to do with a conflict of separation of a sexual nature. For example, a woman wants to be in a stable, loving relationship with a man but keeps being rejected after having intercourse with them. She keeps going in and out of a conflict of separation of a sexual nature, leading to repeated ulceration of the cervix during separation and healing of cervix following sexual union with a sexual partner. The cancer occurs during the repair phase of this conflict of separation.

Keys to Healing

> Healing doesn't depend on what I wish for, hope for, desire, or what I want, but what I do for my healing.
> —Claude Sabbah

Healing requires the accomplishment of four key goals:

1. Resolve the conflict that is at the root of an illness.
2. Have absolute certainty that we can heal and that healing will take place.
3. Understand and accept the inconveniences and challenges of the healing process itself, without creating doubt and without additional stress being created by the healing phase.

4. Be able to let go, rest, laugh, and engage in pleasurable activities that replenish our spirit and our energies.

The Law of Attraction/Creation

In order to understand why we get sick in the first place and how we can improve the odds of healing from our ailments, it is critical to understand the law of attraction and creation and how it comes into play. There are certain characteristics to this law that plays out not just in terms of health but applies to all areas of our lives.

Every idea that we entertain in the mind in the realm of possibilities tends to become reality. In other words, if it is possible, it will become reality. Thoughts are things, and thoughts tend to materialize. If, for instance, we are surrounded by people with certain common health challenges, it may trigger recurring thoughts of those conditions manifesting in us and lead to an increased likelihood of us getting ill. By the same token, if we are stricken by a disease and continuously entertain the idea of overcoming this disease, the likelihood of being cured goes up exponentially.

The likelihood of manifestation or possibility is in direct proportion to the emotion that accompanies it. For example, if overwhelming fear accompanies the thought of becoming ill with a certain serious illness, the chances of that happening increase. On the other hand, if joy and inner peace accompanies the thought of healing from a serious affliction, these more powerful emotions (based on the scale of consciousness) makes healing much more likely.

Imagination tends to trump will. When there is a battle between imagination and will, imagination will always win. Energy always takes the path of least resistance and the act of will requires the application of a lot more sustained energy than imagination. This is the reason why we so often get the exact opposite outcome from what we truly want. Trying to use willpower alone to overcome an addiction, for example, usually ends up in failure; however, if we consistently envision and imagine ourselves free of the addiction and

enjoying life more than ever, the odds of overcoming the addiction is greatly improved.

When the goal is set firmly in place, the subconscious will find the means to realize it. Be careful of what is said in jest; i.e., "I would just die if I got that job" or "if I won the lottery," because the subconscious may link the goal of getting the job or winning the lottery with actual death when the job becomes reality or the lottery is won.

The suggestion will come to fruition only when it is transformed to auto-suggestion; in other words, when it has been transferred to the deepest part of our consciousness. The good news is that a positive or spiritually motivated thought is thousands of times more powerful than a negative thought.

Everything can either be beautiful or horrible, depending on your perspective and the angle from which something is viewed.

Our present reality is the result of our past imaginations. Our future reality is a result of our present imaginations.

Conflict Resolution

1. Identify the triggering and/or the programming event related to the conflict underlying the disease and release the associated negative deep-felt experience.

2. Find a solution to the conflict.
   a. A practical solution that overcomes the conflict.
   b. A change in perspectives or a solution that transcends the conflict, moving beyond it.

Solution "b" is the more powerful of the two. It involves letting go, which involves accepting reality as it is. This involves moving beyond the lived experience, "the absolute," and then transcending the felt experience; in other words, the negative emotions that were

experienced related to the lived experience. Letting go goes beyond forgiveness and is critical to healing.

The Nature of Conflicts Leading to Deep High Stress (DHS)

1. Sudden unexpected deaths in the family.
2. Hospitalizations.
3. Accidents.
4. Family secrets or personal secrets.
5. Sudden life tragedies.
6. Conflicts involving sorrow or anger.
7. Conflicts involving guilt, remorse, or shame.
8. Conflicts involving profound shocks or frights.

In order to heal from any disease, certain beliefs, most of which were discussed earlier in the chapter titled "Erroneous Beliefs" in greater detail, are of great benefit and often essential in order for healing to take place, especially the first five with the sixth being very helpful in order to be at peace with any outcome.

1. I want to heal.
2. I can heal.
3. I will heal (clear belief that illness is curable or that person is capable of healing).
4. I have absolutely no doubts that any illness can be resolved if the underlying conflict is discovered, brought back to full consciousness, and resolved.
5. I deserve to be healthy.
6. I am cognizant of and at peace with the fact that there is for every human being an expiration date to the physical body.

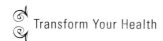

Few of us know when that time will come. There is a point of no return that will come for each of us, when disease progression is such that physical recovery is not possible, or when the physical vehicle simply wears out. Death is not defeat but, ultimately, just one more biological solution. We should not fear death, but should celebrate life, living every day to the fullest, with passion and in love with life. By making peace with death, we are able to live life to the fullest. Healing our wounds not only frees us up to grow and contribute, but sets others free who are carrying our wounds, thereby helping in the healing of not just the individual, but the genealogy.

Important Warnings and Precautions

As discussed previously, the concern about the phenomenon of a healing crisis is very relevant and should not be underestimated. By knowing what might happen when an unresolved conflict is repaired and released, we will be able to act swiftly to help mitigate the symptoms and diseases that might occur during the healing phase. This is one reason why it is important not to discard conventional medicine or overlook its importance. Conventional medicine's forte is the treatment of healing crisis. This is also a critical reason why we should be very cautious about attempting to help others, including loved ones, with the discovery and clearing of their disease-causing unresolved conflicts, unless we have a strong medical background or are well enough educated to avoid the pitfalls inherent to Recall Healing and know when to access the necessary assistance to avoid potential catastrophes.

Heart Disease

Getting in touch with and clearing a major, longstanding conflict of (lost) territory can lead to a myocardial infarction during the healing phase right at the point called the epileptoid crisis (see the Two Phases of Disease diagram on page 138). This is especially true if the conflict was of high intensity and lasted for more than eight months.

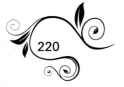

As a matter of fact, the risk is so profound that according to many experienced physicians practicing Recall Healing, Total Biology, or German New Medicine, it is almost a given that this type of person with this severe of a conflict relating to loss of territory may die of a heart attack during the healing phase if strong protective measures are not taken. Such an individual should see a physician, seek medical help to mitigate cardiac risk factors, like high cholesterol, inflammation of the coronaries, or hypercoagulopathy (increased blood clotting tendency), and under medical supervision should consider starting on an aspirin per day immediately. This is especially critical if the person becomes aware that he has this type of conflict and is at a point where he is ready to resolve it.

Brainstem Lesions

When there are tumors in the brainstem or tumor-like effects there from a Hamer Herd (the focus seen on the CT scan of the brainstem associated with emotional conflicts and severe diseases of the kidneys, gastrointestinal tract, pancreas, liver, uterus, or prostate gland), resolution of the conflict can cause a rapid swelling of the brainstem lesion. This swelling can cause the brainstem to herniate through the foramen magnum (opening at the bottom of the skull), which compresses the vital brain centers that control breathing and heart rate. If this condition is not treated quickly with potent diuretics and steroid drugs, the patient often dies.

For additional information on the subject of Recall Healing, go to www.academyCIM.com for online courses on Recall Healing taught by Gilbert Renaud, PhD, and David Holt, DO, HMD. Also visit Gilbert Renaud's Web site recallhealing.com for information on his Recall Healing seminars given around the country.

Basic Steps Toward Optimum Health

Most people are under the false impression that they are destined to suffer health problems no matter what they do and that healing from an especially chronic health problem is not even in the realm of possibility for them. The medical community has done more than its fair share to expand on this myth and has convinced people to see that they are destined for ill health no matter what they do. They might as well get used to the idea of controlling rather than curing disease.

What we have lost perspective of is the fact that the human body has an extraordinary ability to transcend adversity and to heal itself, in spite of the tremendous abuse that it takes. Starting with our lifestyle habits, we abuse our bodies mercilessly with poisonous man-made or heavily processed foods sprayed with pesticides and herbicides, grown in depleted soil, and then wonder why we don't have energy or vitality. The vast majority of us lie around our living rooms staring at a rectangular-shaped object with a device in our hands literally making it possible to sit for hours not having to get up, except to go to the bathroom and get food. We drive around in our fancy cars, attempting to get as close to the entrances of places where we can buy anything imaginable and do many other things in an attempt to minimize the need for physical activity. We avoid the sun like the plague, spend as much of our time as possible indoors, don't even know what water tastes like, and somehow take it for granted that our bodies will just keep on going regardless.

Transform Your Life

This is as much a testimonial of our crimes against our bodies as it is of the extraordinary resilience of the human body to persevere against all odds. The bottom line is that if we can find the motivation to follow a set of basic steps, then almost any chronic or acute illness can be cured, including the most dire of them, like cancer. The first and most important of these steps has already been addressed in the chapter on Recall Healing. We have to discover first and foremost our subconscious, unresolved conflicts that download as disease and dysfunction to the body to allow the conscious mind to be able to stay conscious enough for the survival of the individual. These unresolved inner conflicts also play havoc on our self-awareness, our motivation, and our intuition, making it more difficult to move toward solutions.

This is the primary reason why the vast majority of people fail to succeed in getting their health back, even when they know what to do or at least have a basic idea. Take, for example, obesity. We know through surveys and studies that an average of 95 percent of all people who go on diets of whatever kind and are successful in losing weight regain all of it and more within two years, and 98 percent within five years. It is no wonder, then, that obesity rates are as high as they are, at 33 percent of all adults, with 65 percent overweight. As a matter of fact, when we look at people age twenty-five and older, that rate climbs to an astonishing 80 percent of all Americans with the concomitant skyrocketing incidence of diabetes, hypertension, cancer, heart disease, gallbladder disease, psoriasis, hypothyroidism, chronic fatigue, depression, and so on, and a progressively diminishing quality of life.

The unresolved inner conflicts that lurk within us act as programming that is hard to overcome without a dramatic increase in awareness. This growth and awareness is facilitated when we remember that our outer universe is always a reflection of our inner universe; in other words, in order to rehabilitate our outer shell (the body), we have to heal our inner wounds (our unresolved inner conflicts). As we accomplish this we are more and more likely to succeed at following through with the following basic steps toward optimum

health. Healing unresolved inner conflicts means healing from the top down (the spirit and mind) and also from the bottom up (the physical body). Both have to occur concurrently for us to be successful. In order to gain the necessary physical energy (cell energy) for healing to take place, we have to be successful in reforming our dietary habits, increasing our physical activity, and performing the other basic steps necessary for healing.

Step 1: Eat Your Way Back to Health

When we were growing up, many of us may remember our mothers telling us that we are what we eat, and we better eat our Brussels sprouts, or we risk turning into fertilizer, pushing up daisies well before our time. Our mothers were right to a significant degree. However, you may still ask, "What is healthy, and what is not?" Even in this day and age, there is a considerable amount of confusion and a great amount of disinformation on this topic. This situation is created by special interest groups that are intent on staying as profitable as possible, even at your expense. There is also willful ignorance because so many of us are just too comfortable and don't really want to pay the price for change.

"So what is the best diet?" you may ask. Well, surprise, surprise … there is no one perfect diet for everyone. However, there is one perfect diet for you as an individual. The challenge is finding out what that might be. Your greatest tool is becoming more self-aware and reconnecting with your God-given intuition, which we all have but most have lost track of. There are certain guidelines that I will summarize to help you find your right diet.

Know Your Metabolic Type

There are three possible metabolic types, and each of us is one of those three; i.e., a carbohydrate type, a mixed type, or a protein type. You gauge your type based on how you typically respond in terms of your energy, ability to concentrate, your moods, and general sense

of well-being to meals that are either high in carbohydrates, high in protein, or balanced between the two. If you feel more energetic, have better concentration, have a tendency toward better moods, and have a better sense of well-being on average following meals that are high in fruits, vegetables, and grains, you are more than likely a carbohydrate type. On the other hand, if you tend to get tired, feel irritable, have difficulty concentrating, and just generally don't feel too well after eating this type of meal, especially if it occurs within two hours of eating that meal, you are probably a protein type or a mixed type (or have a food sensitivity to a food that should be good for you).

If you feel all the positive ways listed in the previous paragraph after eating a meal high in protein, including meats, dairy, and/or dry beans with or without vegetables low in the glycemic index, you are probably a protein type or a mixed type. If you feel best when eating a balanced mix of all food categories listed, you are probably a mixed type. It now becomes obvious what you should do based on what metabolic type you are.

If you are a carbohydrate type, you should consume a large percentage of your food as carbohydrates, including low to medium glycemic index vegetables and fruits, as much as 15 percent of your diet as whole grains, some dry beans, and only light, low saturated fats, and animal proteins in small amounts, like chicken, fish, and Cornish hens. Some low-fat or no-fat dairy also may be fine. As a carbohydrate type, it also will be critical for you to eat five to six meals per day, rather than one to two meals per day, which is what most Americans do. If you don't eat more frequently, you will tend to run out of steam within four to five hours, and your metabolism will remain suboptimal.

If you are a protein type, you will tend to do better in terms of your metabolism when you eat a diet richer in protein and fats and lower in carbohydrates. High-protein foods include red meat, chicken, turkey, and fish like salmon. This should be augmented with a lot of low-glycemic index vegetables and low-glycemic index fruits. (See later chapter for glycemic index of foods.) Protein types

should avoid grains and potatoes completely and do well with liberal amounts of healthy fats and oils, like extra virgin olive oil, coconut oil, organic butter, and nuts. Nuts and seeds make good snacks, especially nuts like walnuts or almonds. Protein types are especially vulnerable to alcohol and experience a major energy depletion shortly after drinking.

Mixed types should combine the principles outlined above, but should still be leery of heavy-duty animal proteins, like red meat and dark meats of chicken and turkey, and should eat less grains than carbohydrate types. They also should eat lots of vegetables and more fruit than protein types. They also tend to do better with a little bit more healthy fats in their diet than do carbohydrate types.

Signs that you are eating right:

1. You feel energetic after meals and maintain your energy beyond two hours following a meal.
2. Your head is clear, and concentration is sharp.
3. It is easier to keep a positive disposition.
4. You feel satisfied after meals without being overfull.
5. Food cravings disappear, especially those to sweets.
6. Symptoms of illness tend to improve or at least stay the same.

Signs that you are eating wrong:

1. Your energy is poor or suboptimal and stamina is reduced.
2. You are fuzzy-headed and have a hard time concentrating following meals.
3. It is hard to keep a positive mind-set, and you are more likely to be moody.
4. You continue to feel hungry after meals, even when you eat what should be enough or too much.
5. You crave something sweet and feel dissatisfied after meals.
6. Symptoms of illness tend to worsen or spike.

Know Your Blood Type

This is another defining factor that greatly influences your response to different food choices because there is some correspondence between blood types and metabolic types. For example, blood type O's are more likely to be protein types who do relatively well eating diets higher in animal flesh, except pork, but do not do well when they eat grains, especially wheat and corn. They also fare poorly on most dairy products; starchy vegetables, especially potatoes; and other high-glycemic index carbohydrates. They also cannot tolerate simple sugars very well and should avoid high-glycemic index fruits, such as oranges, cantaloupe, and honeydew melons. They tend to thrive on nuts and seeds, except peanuts and cashews.

Blood type A's tend to be the stark opposite of type O's and are far more likely to be carbohydrate or mixed metabolic types. They are known to be vulnerable to conditions of the stomach and have difficulty making enough acid, especially to digest proteins. They often develop vitamin B12 deficiencies because the stomach does not make enough of a factor called intrinsic factor essential for the absorption of vitamin B12. This also makes them vulnerable to conditions like chronic fatigue; autoimmune diseases, like hypothyroidism; and immune deficiency, with a resultant greater vulnerability to infections. Type A's make great vegetarians, but do not do well consuming a lot of meat. If they do eat any meat, it has to be small amounts and light, low-fat versions usually from smaller animals, like chicken. On the other hand, they do a lot better with most dairy, eggs, and whole grains, except wheat, and do relatively well on most beans and vegetables, except bell peppers, cabbage, potatoes, and sweet potatoes. They do well on most fruits, except subtropical fruits, like bananas, oranges, mangoes, and papaya, and most nuts and seeds, especially peanuts. It is also important for them to limit saturated fats in their diets, and they tend to do much better with more frequent, smaller meals.

Type B's and A-B's tend to do the best on our modern diets and would be more likely to be carbohydrate types or mixed metabolic types than protein types. Both types make great vegetarians because

Transform Your Health

they do not do very well consuming a lot of animal flesh, with the exception of fish. Most poultry, except turkey, is problematic to them, and so is pork. Dairy and eggs also are often beneficial, and they do well with grains, such as oats, rice, millet, and spelt. Wheat and corn are again problematic, and so are a number of nuts, such as peanuts, cashews, and pistachios. They do well with most beans, vegetables, and fruits.

Your blood type also tends to predict which foods you may be allergic to because of lectins associated with your blood type that make your system incompatible with certain foods. For instance, blood type O's have lectin-mediated sensitivities to wheat and other gluten-containing grains, whereas blood type A's have the same for red meat and other heavy animal proteins. For further information on blood types and diets, you can read *Eat Right 4 Your Type*, by Dr. Peter J. D'Adamo.

Know Your Food Sensitivities

Food sensitivities constitute a hidden epidemic that is pervasive in our society, with probably over 90 percent of our population affected and the vast majority not having a clue that they have them or what they are. A much smaller percentage of our population has acute onset allergy reactions to certain foods, and these are easy to identify. There is also a type 1 allergic reaction, which means that symptoms start within seconds or minutes of ingesting the offending food. The vast majority of sensitivity reactions to foods are delayed-type reactions, which can occur as long as seventy-two hours after food is ingested (usually twelve to forty-eight hours). This means that unless you are tracking every food you eat and every meal and closely monitoring symptoms, you will never even suspect that reactions to foods might be stealing your thunder.

A vast array of common maladies are associated with or at least exacerbated by sensitivities to food, including hay fever; recurrent upper respiratory infections; migraines; tension headaches; blurry vision; rashes, such as eczema; psoriasis; dry skin; palpitations; irritable bowel syndrome; constipation; water retention; diarrhea, unex-

Transform Your Life

plained weight gain; chronic fatigue; irritable bladder; and pain syndrome of various kinds, including arthritic pain of the joints or back or muscle, and pain like in fibromyalgia syndrome. More serious conditions that are well-known in the natural medical field to have very strong correlation with food sensitivities and are seen as the key causal factor in many of these include gallbladder disease, like gallbladder stones and inflammation; appendicitis; inflammatory bowel disease, including ulcerative colitis and Crohn's disease; asthma; and even coronary artery spasms, a form of angina.

The five most common allergenic foods in descending order in my practice are cow dairy, wheat, corn, soy, and eggs. Other foods that are often allergenic include cane sugar; peanuts; shellfish; oranges; black pepper; food additives, like artificial sweeteners; preservatives and coloring agents; mustard; coffee; white potatoes; beef; chicken; pork; tomatoes; strawberries; bananas; apples; almonds; walnuts; baker's yeast; brewer's yeast; barley; rye; and oats. Clinical workups for food sensitivities may include the use of bioenergetic testing through EAV technologies and kinesiological testing, and are then correlated with clinical improvements of symptoms and conditions with elimination of the foods that test to be causing sensitivity.

A way that any person can determine if he has a food allergy is with a pulse test. At least four hours after the last food or nutrient ingestion and after sitting quietly in a chair for five minutes, take your pulse rate, eat a single food (for example, an apple or baked chicken without spices or breading or added oils), rest quietly for fifteen more minutes in the chair, and then take your pulse again. If your pulse raises at least fifteen beats per minute after eating that food, compared with the pulse rate before eating, then that food is definitely an allergen. If the pulse raises ten to fourteen beats per minute, then that food may be an allergen.

Within the cow dairy category, milk and cheese seem to be the worst culprits. Dairy may be high in calcium, and we have all been deluged with ads touting dairy's importance in preventing osteoporosis, however, due to the processing, which includes pasteurization (flash heating) and homogenization (where raw milk gets churned

at high speeds to micronize fat particles to avoid cream from separating), calcium gets turned into an inorganic form that is poorly absorbed. Dairy products also tend to acidify the body, causing calcium to move from the bones instead of into the bones. Americans eat more dairy products than most other people in the world, yet Americans have the highest rate of osteoporosis. Countries like Japan and China that consume about one-fifth as much dairy per person have one-fifth the rate of osteoporosis. Is it possible that there may even be a reverse correlation? Unfortunately, this answer will have to wait because the dairy industry certainly will not be funding studies to figure this out.

Wheat, corn, and soy sensitivities are exceedingly common in the United States and seem to be increasing rapidly. The main reason for this might be the fact that the vast majority of corn and soy products here in the United States are now manufactured from GMO (genetically modified organism) sources. We see the same tendency toward food sensitivities in grains, fruits, and vegetables, where genetic manipulation is being employed. Very strange things happen with genetic engineering. Grains, like wheat and corn, often are contaminated with mycotoxins produced by fungi that grow on these crops when stored for lengthy periods of time, especially in humid conditions. A mycotoxin called psilocybin is produced by a mushroom-like fungus that grows on stored wheat and has LSD-like mood-altering effects in humans. This may be one reason why wheat products are so addicting and hard to remove from the diet. Some people's addictions to grains, like wheat, rival those of street drugs to the point where they go through physical withdrawal symptoms when they cannot get their hands on these foods. They usually get irritable, sometimes are manic or anxious; may have palpitations, increased blood pressure, sweating, and increased perspiration; and often have a major drop in energy. They also may have tremors and in certain cases even seizures, especially if they have a previously diagnosed seizure disorder.

Other mycotoxins produced by fungal contaminants on grains include aflatoxin, which is a causative agent in liver cancer and

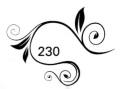

immune dysfunction in animals and humans; zearalenone, which has estrogen-like effects, leading to precocious puberty in prepubescent girls and feminizing changes in males; and ergot-like mycotoxins, which might be contributing to hypertension and neurological problems.

Genetically engineered corn is a cause for great concern, not only because it is so sensitizing, but also because corn and corn byproducts are invading and corrupting our food supply seemingly from top to bottom. It is hard to find a single processed food that doesn't have some form of corn derivative in it, and corn is used on a massive scale as feed for animals whose flesh and byproducts we consume. GMO crops, like corn, consumed by animals impact their health, as they do ours, and when we consume products from these contaminated animals, it adversely affects our health.

Corn byproducts are even found in a large number of supplements in which cornstarch is commonly used as a filler. This includes most of the best-selling multivitamins on the market. Also, certain vitamins, like vitamin C, are almost always derived from corn. It is estimated that as much as 99 percent of vitamin C on the market here in the United States is derived from corn.

High fructose corn syrup has become another huge problem in our food supply. Because it is so much cheaper than cane sugar or beet sugar (it is a byproduct in the manufacturing of corn-based ethanol), food manufacturers prefer to use it rather than cane sugar. All regular soft drinks, most fruit juices, ketchup, mayonnaise, salad dressings, cookies, candies, breads, pastries, and more are sweetened with high fructose corn syrup. At one time, Cuba was the primary source of cane sugar for the United States. Since the boycott of Cuban products started in the 1960s, Americans have been forced to find alternative sources of sweetening agents, such as high fructose corn syrup. With this change, the incidence of obesity and related illnesses really started spiking and is continuing to go through the roof. It is known that very high levels of fructose intake, further complicated by possible sensitivity to its source (corn), increases insulin resistance, which is the underlying mechanism by which

obesity occurs, and its associated long string of illnesses, like adult onset diabetes mellitus, hypertension, high cholesterol, coronary artery disease, cancer, and so on.

It is important to note that any food known to man can be associated with food sensitivity. Not only that, but what you are sensitive to today may not be what you are sensitive to tomorrow. The reason for this is that a larger and larger percentage of our population is developing increased gut permeability (leaky gut syndrome). In other words, the integrity of the intestinal tract mucous membrane gets damaged or disrupted, and instead of the mucous membrane cells being tightly connected by cell bridges, these cell bridges break down, allowing the space for partially digested food particles to leak into the lymphatic system beyond the mucous membrane. The body then is forced to mount a defense against these food particles, especially larger undigested or partially digested protein particles, treating them as invaders that need to be destroyed. This sets off a chain reaction leading to the symptoms and conditions just described.

Factors Contributing to Increased Gut Permeability

1. Poor Food Choices: Processed and man-made foods are dead foods with very little nutrient value. They contain an incorrect ratio of nutrients, lots of toxins, and poisons to boot. These foods do not provide enough nutrition to feed the gut properly, let alone the rest of the body. They have no enzymes, very few usable vitamins or minerals, and provide no vitality.

2. Poor Acid and Enzyme Production: Again, because of poor food choices (foods with none of their own enzymes, allergenic foods causing swelling of the mucous membranes of the stomach and the small bowel and stress on the pancreas), acid production and enzyme production nosedive. The result is that food cannot be properly digested, causing even more stress on the lining of the small bowel and increased gut permeability.

3. Chemicals in Food: Pesticides, herbicides, and fungicides also

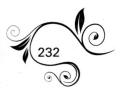

contribute to damage of the intestinal tract and the rest of the body.

4. High Sugar Intake and High-starch Diets: These things contribute to the growth of pathogenic (disease-causing) organisms with further disruptive effects on the stomach, the small bowel, and often the large bowel. Yeast like organisms, such as Candida, parasites, and pathogenic bacteria, thrive in the gut when large amounts of processed carbohydrates and simple sugars are consumed.

5. Microwaved Food or Fluids: Consuming solid foods or fluids cooked or heated in microwave ovens is another major contributor to the epidemic of increased gut permeability that we see these days. A couple of years ago, my daughter Morgan asked me for some ideas for a science project that she had to do for her middle school science class. One of my suggestions was to study the effects of microwaved spring water compared to spring water heated on the stovetop on the growth of plants. I had seen pictures of a similar experiment done by another student a few years earlier where the plant was fed cooled down microwaved water and was dumbfounded by the results then. The plant fed the microwaved water in that experiment died within nine days.

She enthusiastically grabbed onto this suggestion and did her experiment with two small jalapeno plants that were almost exactly the same size at the start of the experiment. She watered one plant every day with microwaved water, cooled down before watering, and the second plant with water heated on the stovetop and cooled down before watering. She gave each plant the same amount of water each day, kept them in the same location outside in the sun, and kept close track of their growth for four weeks.

What happened was very striking to everyone who witnessed her experiment. The first plant, fed water heated on the stovetop, grew rapidly and even had a couple of tiny jalapenos on it by the end of the experiment. The second plant, fed microwaved water, did not grow one bit, and did not produce jalapenos or even one blossom. What was even more frightening (even to the most skeptical teachers and parents) is what happened after the science fair was over.

(By the way, she won first prize and an invitation to participate in the Texas statewide science fair.) Immediately following the conclusion of her school science fair, we transplanted both plants into the same, but much bigger, container and fed both regular, previously unheated spring water. The plant previously given stovetop-heated water grew like wildfire and went on to produce a large number of healthy looking jalapenos. The second plant, previously fed microwaved water, lost all its leaves within three days of transplant and died soon after. My thought was, *Thank God human beings are more resilient than jalapeno plants.* The hypothesis of her experiment had been that microwave radiation can affect the body or a surrogate like a plant in an experiment indirectly when microwave energy is applied at high levels; for example, the water used to water that plant. The hypothesis also includes the possibility that even after the water has cooled down after being microwaved, it still contains electromagnetic energy similar to microwave energy from a microwave oven and will affect living organisms as if they had been exposed to direct microwave energy.

With the sudden dramatic increases in chronic illness around the world, there seems to be a very close correlation between the introduction of microwave ovens into our society and the spike in incidence of chronic disease, such as obesity, heart disease, and cancer. It is unbelievable not that microwaves might truly be dangerous to your health both directly and indirectly, but that almost no research has been published on its possible effects on health. Over 90 percent of American homes and most businesses have microwave ovens, and almost all restaurants, especially fast food restaurants, use very powerful microwave ovens on a large scale. Most people believe that microwave ovens do basically the same thing that heating and cooking food in conventional ovens does. Unfortunately, this is not true. The damage caused by microwave ovens includes a loss of 60 percent to 90 percent of the vital energy content of foods. There is also a marked decrease in the bioavailability (body's ability to utilize the nutrient) of all vitamins and minerals tested. The human body cannot metabolize the byproducts created, including certain

Transform Your Life

amino acids (building blocks of proteins) that become toxic to the human nervous system, affecting memory, concentration, emotional stability, and intelligence. Microwave foods have negative effects on hormone production and increase the number of cancer cells in human blood. This is especially true after prolonged consumption of microwaved food.

6. *Increased Stress:* Even though we are living longer and are statistically safer from threats that plagued our forefathers, we are more stressed out seemingly than ever before, especially in terms of chronic stress. Stress plays a critical role in the disruption of the integrity of the inner lining of the gut through various mechanisms, including higher levels of stress hormones, such as adrenaline and cortisone. There is also decreased production of digestive enzymes and acid production and dysfunction of the smooth muscles that normally propel food through the intestinal tract from top to bottom. This leads to inadequate digestion and elimination, which, in turn, increases exposure to undigested foods, leading to disruption of the gut lining. Parasites that can burrow small holes in our intestinal walls are commonly found in foods we eat. The primary barrier to those parasites establishing residency in the intestine is a normal level of stomach acid, which can kill those food-borne parasites before they pass into the intestine. Chronically stressed people have so much cortisol-induced damage to the stomach cells that produce hydrochloric acid that there is insufficient stomach acid to kill these parasites. It is estimated that 80 percent of visits to doctors are for stress-related conditions. You may think that with all our modern technologies, modern homes, lack of food shortages, abundant water and other essentials for life, relative safety against crime and predators, and living in a country not under siege by an external enemy, we would be relatively stress-free. However, there is abundant evidence that overall stress levels have actually increased through the decades and that it has now mutated from acute stress from time to time, as our ancestors experienced when threatened by predators, warring tribes, natural disasters, and food shortages, to chronic stress, which is potentially with us twenty-four seven, depending on our frame of

mind. With thousands of decisions that have to be made every day and with a steady diet of negative news that is fed to us by the news media, it is no wonder that most of us suffer from stress-related issues. All this stress affects our bodies in many different ways, including disruption of the integrity of the inner lining of the gut.

Glycemic Index of Foods

Another angle on diet and nutrition to be aware of is the glycemic index of foods that you eat; in other words, how quickly that food breaks down to sugar in your intestinal tract and how quickly it is absorbed into the bloodstream. When sugar is rapidly absorbed into the bloodstream, the rapid rise in blood sugar levels leads to a spike in insulin production by the pancreas, which, in turn, causes the liver, muscles, and other cells in the body to absorb this sugar more rapidly from the bloodstream in order to keep blood sugar levels even. This increase in insulin levels and the increase in sugar levels in the cells lead to the increased production of lipids (fats), which contribute to health challenges, such as weight gain. This, in turn, leads to increased insulin resistance, which has been linked to a myriad of chronic health challenges, such as diabetes, hypertension, high cholesterol leading to increased propensity toward heart disease, increased cancer rates, and so forth.

Barry Sears, PhD, who wrote the book *The Zone Diet*, and Dr. Robert Atkins, who wrote the book *The Atkins Diet*, popularized the concept of consuming a diet high in low-glycemic index foods in the 1980s. In order to improve health and lose weight, they both emphasized the role that high-glycemic index foods play in creating excessive insulin production and insulin resistance, which, in turn, leads to numerous common health challenges. It is important if we want to treat health challenges or stay healthy to consume mostly low to moderate glycemic index foods. Even for the healthy, eating large amounts of high glycemic foods, which is what most Americans do, will lead to health problems.

The Standard American Diet (SAD) is generally a high-glycemic index diet also high in saturated, polyunsaturated, and partially

hydrogenated fats. It contains lots of refined carbohydrates, simple sugars, and starchy vegetables, such as white potatoes, in the form of fast foods, like pizza, hamburgers, French fries, other fried foods like chicken and fish, doughnuts, cookies, pasta foods, lots of cheese, milk, lots of soft drinks (regular or diet), tacos, burritos, high starch, high-fat Mexican foods, barbecued meats, lots of bread (especially white bread), luncheon meats, lots of condiments—ketchup, mayonnaise, and mustard—lots of salt and pepper, and don't forget ice cream, cake, pie, and candy. Sound familiar? It is obvious that this diet is anything but low-glycemic index and is a major contributor to the numerous chronic disease epidemics plaguing our society.

The Green Life Diet, which is described below, is the baseline diet that I recommend first to many of my patients, especially when I don't have additional information available on other factors that may need to be taken into account. The Green Life Diet is primarily based on the glycemic index of foods. The Modified Fast and phase 1 of the Green Life Diet contain strictly low glycemic index foods, whereas on phase 2 and 3 of the diet, there is a gradual increase in the amount of higher-glycemic index foods that can be consumed.

The Best Diet

Everyone wants to know what the best diet is for recovery from health problems and for staying healthy. The problem is there is no one best diet that applies to everyone. The Green Life Diet is a good start for the majority of people, but all people are unique and have unique dietary requirements based on a number of factors other than the glycemic index of foods. These other factors include the following:

1. Their overall level of health.
2. The particular health problems they have.
3. Their age and the condition of their teeth, intestinal tract, liver, pancreas, gallbladder, and lymphatic system, associated with the gut.
4. Their metabolic type.

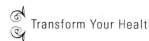 

5. Their blood type.
6. Their food sensitivities.
7. Their level of alkalinity or acidity.
8. The foods that they have available to them in their community or their grocery stores.
9. Their belief systems related to nutrition.
10. Their level of toxicity.
11. Their financial situation and whether or not they can afford to eat a diet that is optimal for their condition.
12. Their social situation and whether or not they have the support of loved ones, health care providers, in-home assistants, or institutional assistants to be able to eat optimally.

The Green Life Diet

The Green Life Diet is a diet that I started using with patients in 1994 when I spearheaded the creation of the Center for Nutrition and Preventive Medicine at the University of Texas Health Science Center at Tyler, Texas. At this location, we treated mostly chronically ill patients with underlying obesity or problems being overweight, and patients who were overweight but otherwise healthy. We had excellent success with patients routinely losing large amounts of weight and with consistent improvements in their associated health challenges. Since 1994, I've treated over ten thousand patients with this diet and continue to have excellent results.

A key part of the success of this diet and other dietary recommendations revolves around behavior modification, which involves changing our way of thinking, discarding erroneous belief systems regarding nutrition and health, and taking on more empowering beliefs. It also requires the discovery of the underlying, unresolved conflicts programming us for the health challenges that we have and the self-defeating health habits that accompany them. This aspect (Recall Healing) has become the most important part of all of my

individualized treatment programs for obesity and other health challenges.

Of course, the success of the Green Life Diet also has been closely correlated not just with improved eating habits, but with increased levels of physical activity and the successful implementation of other basic steps to healing. The 2008 version of the Green Life Diet has a lot of similarities with its original 1994 version, but has had some critical elements added, like metabolic typing, blood typing, and the elimination of foods that we are sensitive to. What is unique about the Green Life Diet is that it emphasizes the fact that every individual is unique and there is no diet that fits all.

We already discussed the importance of figuring out your metabolic type, and there are quite dramatic differences in the ideal food choices for each group. In addition, we discussed the importance of knowing your blood type as additional insights are gained into what food choices will give you the greatest likelihood of optimal health. We discussed the importance of knowing your food sensitivities because these are becoming almost universal and impact everything, including your metabolism and your overall health.

The next aspect of the Green Life Diet is focused on glycemic index and is the main parameter in determining the four phases of this diet including the Modified Fast. It is divided into four phases to correspond with the overall health of the patient and more specifically with the health problems that an individual may have. Each phase is additive, with the Modified Fast a very restrictive low-glycemic index, alkalinizing phase for patients who are very ill or who want to bring about rapid shifts in their health status. It is focused on facilitating detoxification and rapidly reducing insulin production and resistance. Phase 1 is next and is more expansive than the Modified Fast but still focused on strictly low-glycemic index food choices, but with organic animal products added back in. Phase 2 expands food choices further with the addition of moderate-glycemic index foods, and phase 3 adds in small amounts of high-glycemic index foods, such as grains, as long as they are minimally processed and they don't have unhealthful ingredients added, like

table salt, black pepper, sugar, artificial sweeteners, peanut products, canola oil, partially hydrogenated fats, and so on.

The Modified Fast and phase 1 are recommended for the vast majority of individuals suffering from conditions linked to insulin resistance. Insulin resistance means that the body does not respond to the hormone insulin like it should. Insulin is the hormone responsible for facilitating and activating the movement of sugar from the bloodstream into the cells of the body. Insulin resistance is probably the most important mechanism responsible for the development of a wide array of modern-day health challenges, including adult onset diabetes, hypertension, and high cholesterol, and plays a principle role in increasing the risk for most cancers, coronary artery disease, sleep apnea, fatigue, depression, and so many other illnesses that the list would fill a whole page.

Phase 1, when adjusted for metabolic type and blood type, is an extraordinarily effective diet that often brings about rapid improvements in the conditions listed above, especially if food sensitivities also are identified and those foods eliminated. Even cancer patients may experience rapid and dramatic turnaround, especially when the Modified Fast and later phase 1 are combined with juicing, especially of vegetables.

The Modified Fast

The Modified Fast is usually recommended for the first two to six weeks before starting the Green Life Diet phase 1 in patients with serious health problems or those who want rapid improvement to other frustrating health challenges. I see a lot of patients in my office who come to me as a last resort after they have tried everything else or have been referred to me by physicians or other health care providers who just don't know what else to do with these people who have very complex health challenges and who are often taking a smorgasbord of drugs. In these cases, I will recommend the Modified Fast before switching over to the Green Life Diet phase 1.

This diet is an alkalizing vegetarian fast that assists in detoxing the body, improving immune system function, and decreasing

inflammation. It is also a great way to dramatically improve insulin resistance. Most subjects following this protocol will notice a surge in their energy if done properly, but there are some who may feel tired and even achy initially, especially if the body is detoxing too fast. If this scenario arises, the fast may need to be interrupted temporarily and supplemented with other phase 1 food choices; for instance, more beans and some organic animal proteins. In rare instances, some whole grain products may even need to be added in for a day or two to mitigate "die off" reactions or symptoms related to a too rapid detoxification of the body. These may include quinoa, spelt, or buckwheat products. The use of herbal and homeopathic remedies to facilitate gentle detox is also very helpful here and can even be critical to avoid very uncomfortable die off or detox reactions. It is essential when doing the Modified Fast to eat no less than every two to three hours, especially because of the absence of animal proteins and whole grains.

The Modified Fast includes all *low-glycemic index vegetables*. These include all the green leafy vegetables, artichokes, asparagus, brussel sprouts, string beans, green beans, bean sprouts, bamboo shoots, broccoli, cabbage, cauliflower, celery, cucumbers, eggplant, all the different types of lettuce, onions, kale, parsley, pea pods, all colors of bell peppers, spinach, all types of squash, tomatoes, turnips, water chestnuts, watercress, and zucchini. Even though carrots and beets are higher in glycemic index, we do allow some patients to eat and juice them, especially if they are not diabetic or don't have yeast overgrowth. We instruct them to juice at least two times a day and as many as eight times a day for patients with cancer.

This diet also includes all *low glycemic index fruits*. These include avocados, fresh cranberries, cherries, grapefruits, plums, strawberries, blueberries, raspberries, kiwis, blackberries, boysenberries, cantaloupes, lemons, and limes. No canned or dried fruits are allowed. Fresh is preferred, but frozen can be used if fresh is unavailable.

Nuts and seeds are allowed as snacks in between meals. Powdered medical foods manufactured by certain nutraceutical companies for support of specific organ functions or health challenges

also can be used. These do not have any artificial sweeteners, toxic ingredients, soy, dairy, wheat, or corn, but are fortified with rice protein (which is hypoallergenic) and can be taken as a meal by mixing them with water or even making a smoothie out of them by blending them with frozen fruit, for example. It is essential to drink water only spiked with alkalizing lemon, lime, or grapefruit, and herbal teas are also fine, as long as they are caffeine-free.

Cooked dry beans and lentils are acceptable but are limited to small amounts for patients with insulin resistance, including diabetics and those struggling with obesity. Super green foods (like barley green, spirulina, chlorella) are of great benefit when detoxing the body and to support digestive tract health.

It is imperative to include significant amounts of healthy fats, including extra virgin olive oil, extra virgin coconut oil, grape seed oil, sesame oil, and flax oil. Patients are instructed to eat every two to three hours during the day (six meals and snacks per day).

Avoid whole animal products, dairy products, eggs, sugars, sugar substitutes (except xylitol or stevia), starches and grains, vegetable oils, and acidic foods, including vinegar, pickles, pickled olives, pickled onions, and sauerkraut.

During the Modified Fast, it is critical to avoid foods that you are sensitive to. This can be established either through elimination of foods suspected of being sensitizing if adverse reactions occur during the Modified Fast or can be established through bioenergetic evaluation or kinesiology testing, if available.

Phase 1

All foods listed in the Modified Fast are included in phase 1.

Most vegetables are included in phase 1, except starchy vegetables, like potatoes (especially white potatoes), and moderate to large amounts of sweet potatoes, winter squash (acorn, butternut), and green peas. Also limit the intake of cauliflower and sweet veggies, like carrots and beets, especially in cooked or juiced form. Raw cauliflower, carrots, beets, and cooked sweet potatoes and winter squash are acceptable in smaller amounts but need to be used carefully in those with diabetes or yeast overgrowth. Dill or sour pickles are generally acidifying but acceptable in small amounts on occasion as part of phase 1.

Fruits should be limited to low-glycemic index fruits, especially in those dealing with insulin resistance; for example, those with frank diabetes and those with yeast overgrowth. Ideal fruits include grapefruits, lemons, limes, avocados, plums, figs, kiwis, strawberries, blackberries, raspberries, and most other berries, especially fresh. Dried fruit tends to have a slightly higher glycemic index, compared with fresh fruit. Green apples, like Granny Smith apples, slightly green pineapples, slightly green bananas or plantain bananas, pears, cantaloupes, and honeydew melons are acceptable, again, except in those with frank diabetes, excessive acidity or yeast problems. Another fruit that fits into this category and that many forget is a fruit are olives. Black and green olives are both valuable because of their high omega-9 (mono unsaturated) fatty acid content.

Dry beans cooked into soups or stews are generally acceptable, except beans high in starch, like black-eyed peas, lima beans, and kidney beans. Those dealing with excess weight or insulin resistance should eat beans only in moderation. Certain types of beans are contraindicated for certain blood types. Those with protein-type metabolisms do well consuming larger amounts of beans, whereas those with carbohydrate-type metabolisms less so.

Nuts and seeds are generally low glycemic index, except peanuts and cashews, which should be avoided. Pistachios and macadamia nuts are also not ideal in significant amounts as part of phase 1.

Other nuts and seeds, on the other hand, are a very important part of the phase 1 diet and are especially handy as snacks, especially almonds and walnuts. Excessive amounts of nuts and seeds, though, are not appropriate during this phase because of the relatively high calorie concentrations. Be very careful that they are fresh. Nuts easily go rancid and ideally should be kept refrigerated after opening a container of them, especially if they are going to be kept for more than a few days before being consumed. Freshly ground flax seed, up to one to two tablespoons per meal, is also a very good source of fiber and omega-3 fatty acids.

In addition, phase 1 also includes meats, strictly organic; i.e., range-fed, including lean beef, buffalo, lamb, veal, rabbit, venison, turkey, chicken, duck, ostrich, emu, or goose. Always trim visible excess fat from meats and skin off poultry. Bake, broil, or sauté in extra virgin olive oil or extra virgin coconut oil only. Avoid all highly processed meats. Limit red meat intake (even blood type O's) to no more than one to two small portions a week. Type A's should avoid red meat entirely. Carbohydrate types should still focus mainly on vegetables, fruits, nuts and seeds, and beans, and far less on animal products, whereas protein types should consume more foods high in protein content, such as beans, bean sprouts, nuts, and seeds, and should be able to consume more animal products if they choose to. Mixed types will find themselves somewhere in between, needing both high-carb choices and high-protein choices.

Most fresh fish is good, depending on your blood type, especially ocean fish, with limited amounts of freshwater fish. Avoid bottom-dwellers, like catfish, and the large predator fish of the ocean, like tuna, swordfish, shark, and mackerel. If you can find absolutely clean sources of shellfish, they may be okay to add to your diet; however, most sources are not very clean, and as the scavengers of the ocean, they are almost always contaminated with higher levels of heavy metals, pesticides, solvents, PCB's and other man-made poisons. Again, you can broil, bake, or sauté, but avoid the skin. Avoid anything breaded and fried.

Extra virgin olive oil, grape seed oil, almond oil, sesame seed oil, and other nut oils make good salad dressings when combined with organic cider, wine vinegar, lemon juice, or lime juice. Avoid canola oil, peanut oil, and other vegetable oils. Choose oils that are not bottled in plastic. Get your salad dressings in glass bottles when at all possible. Plastic residues leak out of plastic bottles even more readily when filled with oil than with water.

Use limited organic butter only. No margarine, buttermilk, sour cream, ice cream, or yogurt. Use limited amounts of no-fat or low-fat cheese, like string cheese, mozzarella cheese, feta cheese, and low-fat cottage cheese.

Eggs are included in this phase but eat strictly organic, preferably soft-poached or soft-boiled eggs. Egg yolk contains cholesterol, but it is not the cholesterol that hurts you. It is when the cholesterol is oxidized, like when eggs are hard-fried or hard-boiled, that it hurts you. Scrambling eggs is the worst because it oxidizes even more of the cholesterol.

Filtered or spring water is preferred. Add a slice of lemon or lime to your water to alkalinize it. Limit coffee intake, and strictly organic coffee should be used. Coffee is one of the most pesticide-laden crops in the world in its regularly cultivated form. Stevia and xylitol are the only sweeteners to be used. Honey may be okay in small amounts. Herbal teas are also good. Green tea and even regular unsweetened tea is good. Use regular tea in moderation. Avoid all artificial sweeteners, except the ones listed. Splenda, NutraSweet, and aspartame are the most poisonous.

One of the big challenges that people have with eating healthy is that they frequently equate it with food boredom. Most people have the idea that eating healthy means eating a bland, boring, simplistic diet. But fortunately, that is not true. I would say that it's rather critical that we be innovative by flavoring foods adequately with healthy seasonings and by varying the food choices that we make. Even though there are some restrictions on the food choices contained in a healthy diet, there are still a very large number of food choices that can be made.

Seasoning of food is not only excellent for spicing up your culinary universe, but also can have its own unique health benefits. A vast number of commonly used condiments have been found to have unique health benefits. Unprocessed, unbleached sea salt, for example, is rich in trace minerals and can be used to boost energy production in many people suffering from chronic fatigue. This also applies to those with weak adrenal glands and many who have an intolerance to stress. This, however, is not true about regular, processed table salt, which is poisonous to the human. It has been interesting to me to note that unprocessed sea salt seems to have very little, if any, detrimental effect on people suffering from high blood pressure, whereas processed table salt is clearly counterproductive for a large percentage of hypertensives. There are entire books written on the health benefits of sea salt, and it is certainly a topic worth exploring further. Use strictly naturally unprocessed sea salt, like Celtic sea salt.

Other seasonings, like cilantro, cinnamon, parsley, cloves, curry, rosemary, and garlic, have well-described and well-known health benefits. The vast majority of herbal seasonings (like curry, garlic, and cloves) used in the culinary art have been shown to benefit digestion and to reduce the incidence of foodborne illnesses in certain cases. Again, whole books have been written about seasonings and their benefits. Most important here is to make the point again that by spicing up our foods, we not only make food more fun, but can also help ourselves health wise.

It is very helpful in this phase to avoid all grains, starches, and sugars; in other words, all high-glycemic index and even some of the medium-glycemic index foods. This helps to normalize insulin response in individuals with insulin resistance or excess insulin production. Dairy products are limited to a large degree during this phase because they are so acid- and mucus-forming. Wheat, other refined grain products, and dairy products all tend to cause the formation of a mucus layer in the intestinal tract that diminishes the capacity of the small bowel to absorb nutrients. This slime tube is literally like a hose pipe within a hose pipe. Besides interfering with nutrient absorption, it also forms an ideal hideout for bugs

Transform Your Life

and parasites that are all too happy consuming the micronutrients that are not getting to the mucous membrane to be absorbed. These critters also include fungus, like Candida, and pathogenic (disease-forming) material, like E. coli, and they also produce toxins that are absorbed into the lymphatic system around the gut and then into the bloodstream.

This slime tube can be dislodged through the consumption of healthy non-mucus-forming foods and certain supplements that will be described in the next section, and certain mechanical tools, like colema treatments or colema-type irrigations of the large bowel. Colemas are different from standard colonics in that they can be done at home with the right equipment, are gravity-based systems, and are safe, especially when certain basic instructions are followed. If you do decide to order a colema board, make sure you get a list of instructions that are easy to follow so that you don't injure yourself.

Other foods to avoid during this phase include high-glycemic index fruit, like tropical fruits, including ripe bananas, mangoes, and very ripe pineapples. People with frank diabetes with blood sugars that are out of control may also have to minimize these as well as other sweet fruits, like peaches, nectarines, grapes, the sweeter category of apples, watermelon and honeydew. I am not too overly fixated on eliminating these fruits, even in phase 1, unless someone has uncontrolled diabetes or severe yeast overgrowth. It certainly is by far better to eat a balanced diet with a lot of vegetables as part of it, but for those who are just starting to reform their lifestyles, adding fruit is a great first step. Even though fruits are relatively high in sugar and often contain chemicals like pesticides, they still have a lot more good in them than processed foods. When you eat a candy bar or a piece of bread, you are eating a dead food with a very low vitality rating, whereas, the average fresh fruit has a much higher vitality rating and is also filled with enzymes that are essential for health. I do find that people who eat too many fruits and not enough vegetables and other foods tend to run out of energy more quickly and have to eat a lot more frequently. Most fruits tend to alkalinize; however, the fruits high in sugar may actually acidify the body.

Whether fruits are organic or nonorganic also makes a big difference. Nonorganic fruits, especially the thin skin fruits like peaches, nectarines, and plums, average three or four different pesticides in and on them. The problem is that the body has to expend so much energy detoxing these poisons that very little energy is left from these foods for other bodily functions. The more pesticides that are consumed, the more acidic the body also gets.

Black pepper should be avoided because it has no nutritional value, is an irritant to the intestinal tract, and is a common allergen. Ketchup needs to be avoided during this phase of your diet due to its high sugar content. Mustard and mayonnaise should also be avoided during this phase of your diet.

Phase 2

Include all the Modified Fast and phase 1 foods, plus the following.

Phase 2 of the Green Life Diet consists of the addition of moderate-glycemic index foods to the diet and is appropriate for those with significant metabolic diseases that have responded well to the Modified Fast and to phase 1. For example, in someone with frank diabetes whose blood sugars have normalized and who has been able to come off his medications, or the person who was one hundred pounds overweight and has lost fifty to sixty of those pounds, or the hypertensive patient whose blood pressure has normalized off medications may expand his diet to include phase 2 foods. Phase 2 foods also may be appropriate for those dealing with significant metabolic diseases that are not completely under control, but who are doing everything else right, have been on phase 1 for at least six weeks, and are willing to control the portions of these phase 2 foods. This would include certain berries that are medium glycemic index, like blueberries, boysenberries, and cherries, because of their high antioxidant levels, and pineapples because of their high anti-inflammatory enzyme levels (bromelain). Papaya also may be an exception because of its high papaya enzyme content, which is good for digestion. These are all certainly appropriate for level 2. Green, slightly sour-tasting apples also may be eaten as part of phase 1 in most

instances, even though they belong to the medium-glycemic index category. However, the sweeter red varieties should be consumed only as part of phase 2.

Phase 2 foods include larger amounts of vegetables, such as sweet potatoes, winter squash (acorn, butternut), tomato puree, rutabaga, and Jerusalem artichoke. Jerusalem artichoke flour can be used to bake bread as part of this phase, and many health food supermarkets carry bread made from this vegetable. White potatoes in baked or scalloped form are medium glycemic index, but mashed white potatoes are high glycemic index. French fries should be avoided, even though they are medium glycemic index because they are just pure poison. Beans like lima beans, black-eyed peas, and kidney beans can be consumed in smaller amounts during this phase as well.

Moderate-glycemic index grains like quinoa, amaranth, buckwheat, spelt, corn on the cob (non-GMO only), slow-cooked steel-cut oatmeal, wild rice, and brown rice are all in this category and can be consumed if no yeast overgrowth problems remain and in diabetics if blood sugar is well-controlled on diet alone with the patient off all medications; however, these should all be limited to smaller amounts.

Fruits like fresh apricots, peaches, nectarines, blueberries, boysenberries, ripe pineapples, bananas, cantaloupes, honeydew melons, all apples, pears, grapes, and kiwi also can be enjoyed as part of this phase, even though some of them, like grapes, are technically high-glycemic index fruits; however, the types of fruit sugars in these fruits pose less of a problem than those fruits in the third phase of the Green Life Diet.

Unsweetened grapefruit juice, tomato juice, pomegranate juice, and cranberry juice diluted with water to a minimal ratio of one-to-one can be consumed during this phase, but should be limited to eight ounces per day. Other fruits in this phase and in phase 1 also can be juiced but should always be diluted no less than one-to-one and as high as five parts of water to one part of juice.

People in phase 2 should still avoid wheat and wheat byproducts; corn and corn byproducts; processed grains, like oats, barley,

and rye; simple sugars; and tropical fruits, like oranges, orange juice, and mangoes.

Phase 3

Include all the Modified Fast and the Green Life Diet phase 1 and 2 foods, plus the following in moderation.

Phase 3 for those who are in relatively good physical health and at a relatively healthy body weight and who want to maintain or even improve their health, and also for those with metabolic diseases, such as obesity, hypertension, diabetes, and other chronic illnesses, who are fully or almost fully recovered. The foods included in this phase are in some ways a repeat of those in phase 2, with some additions. You even will recognize some of these from phase 1, where small amounts of them were allowed. These can be consumed in larger amounts during this phase, and included are higher amounts of the following: beets, lima beans, carrots, corn on the cob, parsnips, peas, black-eyed peas, red potatoes, white potatoes, sweet potatoes, yams, and chickpeas. These should all either have been eliminated during phase 1 or at least severely restricted and should have been restricted during phase 2.

Fruits now unrestricted include bananas, melons (watermelon, honeydew), mulberries, mangoes, oranges, papayas, pears, and tangerines (fresh or frozen). Again, some of these were mentioned in phase 1 and especially 2, but in phase 3, they can be consumed in a more unrestricted manner. Bread and cereals: fresh stone-ground whole-grain breads, limited to one slice per day with just about any grain except GMO grains and grains known to be stored routinely for many months in silos where they get contaminated with fungus. Acceptable grain products would include some grains already mentioned in phase 2 with some additions: steal-cut oats, barley, millet, spelt, buckwheat, Kamut, quinoa, amaranth, rye, non-GMO corn and wheat, brown and wild rice, and whole-grain crackers with no partially hydrogenated fats. The breads listed above will not be found on regular store shelves, but only in the refrigerated section. This is because partially hydrogenated fats and other preservatives

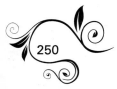

are not present in these foods. Corn should be avoided in America because of the GMO problem here and the fact that the food industry does not have to label foods as derived from GMO sources. In other words, you don't know, and it is, therefore, safer just to stay off of it. Genetic modification makes it much more allergenic than their natural non-GMO counterparts. Use very limited amounts of pasta and strictly whole-grain pasta or pasta derived from other sources, such as spinach.

Fruit juices of different kinds, including orange juice, apple juice, apple cider, and pineapple juice, can be used as part of phase 3, but need to be unsweetened and diluted with water by a one-to-one ratio at a minimum. The ideal is to do freshly juiced fruit juices because of the increased nutrient content and the vitality rating. The maximum is four to eight ounces per day and less for children.

Cashews, popcorn with non-GMO corn, and small amounts of raw honey may be consumed during this phase.

Again, a reminder to be aware of restrictions of any of the foods listed in the Green Life Diet based on blood type, metabolic type, and food sensitivities. Also, remember to eat organic as often as possible, especially in the case of health problems.

Food Combining Rules for the Green Life Diet

1. Eat fruits alone, preferably for breakfast or for snacks, no less than thirty minutes before a meal or three hours after a meal containing other fruits. The exception is vegetables. Other fruits and low-glycemic index vegetables can be consumed together. Fruits and vegetables do not need stomach acid for digestion, whereas foods high in protein do require high levels of acid production in the stomach. If you eat fruits with animal proteins, you create a stalemate in the stomach, with the fruits being digested very slowly and ending up fermenting in the stomach, whereas the digestion of

Transform Your Health

animal proteins also is inhibited because of the alkalinizing effect of the fruits.

2. If you eat cereals for breakfast, also avoid fruits at the same time.

3. Vegetables and, if appropriate for your health, starches and grains, can be consumed together.

4. Never eat animal-source proteins within three hours of starches. So much for meat and potatoes, pizza with meat, pasta with meat, hamburgers, hot dogs, and so on. Animal-source proteins include fish, poultry, eggs, dairy products, beef, and pork. Starches would include foods like potatoes, rice, pasta, crackers, and bread.

5. Avoid eating heavier animal proteins, like red meat or pork for lunch unless your metabolic type or blood type diet recommends it.

6. If you don't know your metabolic type, the best animal-source protein is fish, the second-best is chicken, and third-best is turkey. Red meat and pork are hard to assimilate, except the most resilient O blood type with great stomach acid production. People who are blood type B do better on turkey than chicken.

7. Animal-source proteins combine well with low-glycemic index vegetables, but not with starchy vegetables, like potatoes.

8. Rotate foods so that they are eaten no more often than every three to four days in order to reduce the likelihood of developing food sensitivities.

I frequently hear people say that they know what they are supposed to be eating, but they cannot overcome the cravings for the foods that they are not supposed to eat. As a matter of fact, most people equate dieting with dying and with a reduced quality of life, so much so that the vast majority of people fail in their efforts to make these essential dietary lifestyle changes. In order to understand why it is so difficult for most of us to make long-term changes, we need to realize that most people equate dieting with deprivation. Diets don't

Transform Your Life

work when certain unresolved inner conflicts are present. Just like all illnesses are related to unresolved inner conflicts, so are all dysfunctional lifestyle issues.

Dysfunctional Lifestyles and Unresolved Inner Conflicts: The Story of Pat

Let's take the example of Pat M., who was sexually abused from the time that she was seven years old until she was eleven by an uncle who used to babysit her. Her subconscious conflict became one of not being able to trust men because of her subconscious fear of being abused again and being used as a sexual object. The conflict expresses itself by making her "bigger" in order to protect herself and "to make her less attractive" to men so that she is less likely to be attacked or abused sexually.

Pat also had a conflict of "abandonment" from both her mother and father. Her father abandoned her mother soon after she conceived when he found out that Pat's mom was pregnant and didn't want to deal with it. Therefore, she was born with a partial conflict of annihilation. This conflict also can lead to a tendency toward excessive weight gain, a conflict that expresses itself as follows: "I need to be bigger so that my father who has abandoned me will be able to find me and see me."

Pat also felt abandoned by her mother, who failed to protect her against the sexual abuse that she had experienced at the hands of her uncle. Her mother had a lot of guilt when Pat was a little child because of her short temper and her lack of patience, which caused her to lash out verbally at Pat quite frequently. She allayed her guilt each time by giving Pat candy and other sweet things. Subconsciously, Pat started equating sweets with motherly love. Sweets became a surrogate for her mother's love from early on, continuing into adulthood. Pat was totally unaware of these conflicts that she was harboring at the core of her being.

In addition, Pat had a conflict of self-image, affirmed every time she looked in her bathroom mirror. As a matter of fact, any mirror

that she would look into, solicited or unsolicited, would give her the soul-destroying message "You are fat. Fatso. You have no self-discipline. You have no will power. No one wants you. Everyone thinks you're ugly."

Add to that the mass consciousness around the problem of obesity in our country where women think they are fat even when they are not, where women equate beauty with thinness and ugliness with fatness, where more and more people are now starting to deal with chronic illnesses like diabetes, cancer, and heart disease that has been so strongly linked to obesity and the fact that Pat, as a previously unconscious member of our society, bought into this mass consciousness, you can understand why she was doomed to be fat forever until she became aware of her wounds and unresolved conflicts.

When Pat started seeing me, she weighed 240 pounds. She lost sixty pounds within the first year with me and has kept it off for the past five years. She had a number of associated health challenges, including diabetes, high blood pressure, high cholesterol, hypothyroidism, arthritis in both knees, gastroesophageal reflux disease (hiatal hernia), and a host of other minor ailments. These have all resolved since Pat started her quest to identify and clear the conflicts linked to her obesity and with each one of these maladies.

Pat is representative of millions of patients who have similar life stories and similar challenges and are constantly failing in their attempts to win the battle of the bulge. In my practice, I've seen hundreds of similar success stories over the past decade. The results have continued to get better as my understanding of these underlying conflicts has grown and as I have become more able to help my patients discover them and clear them more efficiently. I have seen patients lose as much as 150 pounds without the aid of radical procedures like stomach bypass surgery, liposuction, or the use of drugs, and have kept it off over a period of more than five years, which is usually the threshold for the definition of long-term success.

Supplements

Because of modern agriculture methods, which tend to leave the soil depleted of almost all trace minerals, the quality of even the healthiest vegetables and fruits and other foods is steadily diminishing. It is estimated that the average fruit or vegetable today, grown under regular agriculture conditions, has as little as one-fifth of the nutrient concentration (vitamins, minerals, antioxidants, and enzymes) of produce grown one hundred years ago. This means that you have to consume up to five times as much of this produce to achieve the same nutrient levels as your ancestors did one hundred years ago. Unless you are grazing all day long and eating mountains of fresh fruits and vegetables or consuming strictly organic freshly picked vegetables and fruits, then you might need to take extra steps to assure adequate nutrient consumption. This is where supplementation can be very helpful as long as the supplements consumed are of high quality and the right type.

Useless or Even Dangerous Supplements

I am convinced that as much as 90 percent of the supplements sold in grocery and health food stores are at best unhelpful and at worst disease-promoting. The reason why I say this is that most manufacturers that make supplements use ingredients, for instance, in multiple vitamins, that are downright poisonous. For example, dl-alpha-tocopherol (the synthetic form of vitamin E) has been shown in studies not only not to help in conditions such as coronary artery disease, but in many cases, to have the potential to make things worse. Even using the natural form of vitamin E (d-alpha-tocopherol) is not nearly as helpful and may even be harmful in the treatment of conditions like coronary artery disease, but the broad spectrum form of vitamin E in the form of tocotrienols, especially the delta and gamma tocotrienols, have been shown to be very helpful in mitigating vascular disease and other maladies.

Another prime example of a problem that we see all over the supplement market is the form that vitamin C comes in. When vita-

min C was studied by Linus Pauling and others twenty to thirty years ago, it was shown to be very helpful in treating malignancies, and there was lots of anecdotal evidence that it made a difference in the treatment of colds and flu and upper respiratory infection. However, something has happened because the latest research over the last few years has shown very little or no benefit from vitamin C. What is critical to note, though, is that the source that vitamin C is derived from has changed and is now made from corn about 99.9 percent of the time. In America, corn used in manufacturing products such as vitamin C is almost 100 percent from GMO corn sources. GMO corn is highly sensitizing, causing people who are sensitive to corn, which may be as high as 80 percent, to get very little, if any, benefit from vitamin C derived from this source. These sensitivities are mostly delayed-type sensitivities, which are very hard to diagnose because of mostly vague, nonspecific symptoms.

By the way, even if you read the small print, in the vast majority of cases, you would not know that most vitamin C is derived from corn. The only time you can be sure it's not from corn is when it specifically states that it is non-corn-based or specifically states that it is made from another source, such as rose hips, cassava, beets, acerola cherry, potatoes, or tapioca.

Natural Is Always Better

Every vitamin and every supplement is either derived from certain plants, other natural sources, or is synthetically made. Only vitamins, minerals, amino acids, and enzymes from the most pristine natural sources can be trusted to deliver some benefit.

Another factor that defines whether a supplement may help you or hurt you is how it is manufactured and packaged. Even if the active ingredients are good for you, fillers, coloring agents, preservatives, and/or flavoring agents can destroy the benefit that would otherwise be derived from a supplement. Far too often, one will see ingredients like cornstarch, artificial sweeteners, maltodextran (corn-derived), and dyes used as ingredients in supplements.

Transform Your Life

Another form of contamination that occurs with a large number of manufacturers is the fact that one machine may be used to encapsulate many different supplements or to make tablets of many different supplements. When these machines are cleaned in between batches, they are often cleaned with solvents, which may not be completely washed off the equipment before the next batch is made, therefore contaminating the next batch of product made with that machine.

Omega-3 Fatty Acids, including fish oil or flaxseed oil, have been shown to be beneficial in the treatment of a number of disorders, including arthritis, coronary artery disease, hypertension, and hyperlipidemias (high blood fats), but unfortunately, the majority of products found in today's marketplace are contaminated to a greater or lesser degree with substances like heavy metals. Some examples are mercury, cadmium, and PCB's. A small handful of companies use strictly uncontaminated fish sources to make their products from and often take additional measures like cold filtering to remove any contaminants that may be present. These products naturally cost more than the products derived from cheaper, but contaminated, sources.

There are many books that can be referenced for more information on supplementation, but I will briefly summarize some of the most useful in the general population, especially for those who are relatively healthy and are interested in prevention more than a cure. For those with significant health challenges, it may be necessary to gather additional information on what supplements might be helpful for specific illnesses. There are forms of bioenergetic testing available, including applied kinesiology, dowsing, and EAV technology (electronic acupuncture by Voll) that may be invaluable when used by trained practitioners. Dowsing is also a technique that can be learned for self-testing, but is only effective if the one using this tool is totally neutral to the results and is in touch with their intuition. One form of dowsing that can be learned is what is called the lean test, which requires one to stand with feet slightly apart in a totally balanced, neutral position, not leaning forward or backward at all. You then take a remedy that you want to test with one hand

and place it over your heart energy center (middle of the chest) or over your solar plexus energy center (over the solar plexus—upper stomach in middle under rib cage). You then silently ask the question "How does my body feel about this?" Or you make an affirmative statement like, "My body needs this." If you feel like you are being pushed backward, the subconscious may be responding in a negative way. If you lean forward, the subconscious may be responding in a positive way. You may enhance the results that you get with this technique by practicing with things that you know are poisonous or beneficial to you.

Applied kinesiology works in a similar way, but requires a second individual. Again, it takes a very high level of integrity and somebody who is skilled in this technique, who knows how to balance an individual before he is formally tested. The term used in applied kinesiology is open regulation, which means that the body is in normal polarity configuration. In other words, the body's south pole is in the right place, and the body's north pole is in the right place, just like a bar magnet. There are numerous factors that can affect open regulation.

Supplements That Make Sense in Sickness and in Health

Multivitamin supplements are probably a good idea for most people to consider taking to fortify the nutrients that they get from food. Again, ensure that you are taking just the highest-quality multivitamin with the highest-quality ingredients or get recommendations from a neutral party that is well-versed in the best products available. Some of the most popular multivitamins on the market that are heavily advertised on television and in print media are not only useless, but may actually damage your health because of the poisonous ingredients used. It is interesting to note that most of these are manufactured by drug companies that are great at presentation, advertising, and marketing, but not as great in terms of their integrity and ensuring that no harm will come from their products.

A good multi-mineral is also helpful in a large percentage of individuals. For example, most Americans don't get enough magne-

sium in their food supply. Ironically, a great emphasis is placed on calcium supplementation, even though the incidence of magnesium depletion far exceeds that of calcium.

This is not meant to be an exhaustive list of possible nutrient deficiencies, but only looks at those nutrients that are deficient in a very large percentage of our population. Other nutrients that may need to be supplemented that are often deficient include:

Anybody living under significant stress may benefit from taking a complex of *B vitamins*. The body needs a lot more of these essential nutrients when under stress to work optimally.

A lot of foods are now fortified with *folic acid* because of its critical importance at preventing certain birth defects. Unfortunately, the folic acid added to cereals and in other foods is not absorbed efficiently and in high enough doses to adequately protect against birth defects. A good multivitamin with folic acid may be sufficient for most people; however, in women who may get pregnant or are thinking about getting pregnant, I strongly recommend an additional 800 micrograms or more above and beyond the minimum dose of 400 micrograms per day.

If you eat a diet high in freshly picked organic vegetables and fruits, you probably don't even need to bother taking *vitamin C*. But if you are in the shoes of the vast majority of our population, not eating healthy and under significant stress, you can do with an extra gram or two of non-corn-based vitamin C. Besides improving your immune system function, there are dozens of other good reasons to take a little extra. If your system is too acid, take a buffered form of vitamin C, and if it's on the alkaline side, take the ascorbic acid form. (See section on alkaline-acid balance.)

The list of reasons to take extra *vitamin D* every day is growing by leaps and bounds. Originally, it was thought to mainly affect the bones, but now it is known to be essential in protecting against a number of malignancies. It is also very helpful in preventing and treating high blood pressure. There are a slew of other reasons why vitamin D is important that will not be dealt with here. Suffice it to say that the average adult, especially those working or living indoors

and getting minimal sun exposure, should take a minimum of 2,000 IUs of the active form of vitamin D (vitamin D-3). Much higher doses than that may be recommended under a supervised setting.

In an era where we are being bombarded by toxicity in our food and in our environment, antioxidants, such as *vitamin E,* are essential for maintaining health. Again, the list of benefits of vitamin E is a mile long, but it is critical to take the right form of it. The most beneficial form of vitamin E is the tocotrienols, which should be taken as a mix of all four types (alpha, beta, delta, gamma tocotrienols). A dose of 400 to 800 IUs is probably sufficient for most.

Vitamin K is also deficient in most people because of our diets and because of generalized gastrointestinal dysbiosis (abnormal growth patterns of bacteria and other organisms in the gut). Vitamin K is one of many nutrients that are made by new bacteria in the intestinal tract. Vitamin K2—as the MK4 and the MK7 form—are the two most valuable forms and are critical in promoting bone health, normal clotting mechanisms, brain health, and cancer prevention.

The vast majority of Americans are deficient in *omega-3 fatty acids* because our diets have become more and more depleted. This is in large part due to the unbalanced diet being fed to animals that we as humans consume. The ideal ratio of omega-6 to omega-3 fatty acids is estimated to be 2-to-1. In America today, the ratio is anywhere from 26-to-1 to as high as 56-to-1, depending on which communities are scrutinized. Essential fatty acids are essential for life, and these kinds of imbalances would obviously have a highly adverse effect on everyday health. The best source for omega-3 fatty acids is fish oil, which contains eicosapentaenoic acid (EPA) and docosahexaenoic acid (DHA). Other sources, such as flax seed oil, contain alpha-linolenic acid that has to be converted in the body to EPA and DHA. In those with good health, this happens efficiently. But in those with poor health, it happens very inefficiently. Omega-3's are essential for everything from normal brain function and nerve function to joint function, cardiovascular function, and even skin function. The benefits are almost endless. Unless you eat

Transform Your Life

ocean-raised fish at least two times a week, you can probably benefit by taking two to three grams of fish oil daily.

Omega-6 fatty acids in our diet: one particular form called gamma-linolenic acid (GLA), is often deficient. This essential fatty acid is critical in the prevention and treatment of inflammation in the body, including the joints and gut. Three commonly used sources for GLA include evening primrose oil, borage oil, and black current seed oil. A dose from one to two grams per day may be helpful to those struggling with inflammation that does not subside when taking just omega-3 fatty acids.

As mentioned before, *magnesium* deficiency may be more of a problem than calcium deficiency. This is especially true for those eating the Standard American Diet (SAD) high in processed foods. Again, a whole book can be written on this mineral alone and its critical importance to overall health. It is critical in the treatment of everything from chronic fatigue and fibromyalgia to osteoporosis and asthma, but one hundred other conditions could be listed. The usual dosage for supplementation is 200 to 600 milligrams per day with the best, most well-absorbed forms being magnesium malate, magnesium glycinate, 2-AEP magnesium and magnesium citrate.

Potassium deficiency is very common due to our diets. By massively increasing fresh vegetable and fruit intake, this deficiency can be quickly eliminated in most individuals. Many with uncontrolled hypertension, diabetes, and fatigue may benefit from potassium supplementation. Those on certain medications, like certain blood pressure medications, should take extra potassium only under medical supervision.

Other minerals, like zinc, copper, selenium, chromium, molybdenum, and nutrients such as coenzyme Q10 and alpha lipoic acid (in the form of R lipoic acid), are often deficient and often helpful to supplement. Do some reading on the conditions that you suffer with, and you may get some good leads on what else might be helpful. For many, the most efficient way to take supplements is under medical guidance and with some form of bioenergetic testing to figure out what is most essential in order to regain your health.

It is estimated that about 95 percent or more of Americans are deficient in *iodine*. The reasons for this include severe soil depletion and, therefore, generalized iodine deficiency in our soil-grown foods, and the fact that seafood consumption in America is much lower than in other countries like Japan where iodine deficiency is much less common. This is further exacerbated by the fact that bromine is used as a preservative instead of iodine in refined grain flour like wheat and corn and because of fluoride and chlorine in our water. These are all halogenous elements that compete with iodine for inclusion in critical functional molecules in the body. The fact that table salt is iodized does not help very much because table salt is poisonous because of the caking agents and bleaching process that it goes through during processing. Its bioavailability is relatively low.

Iodine deficiency contributes to a whole host of illnesses, including low thyroid (hypothyroidism); diseases of the breast, including fibrocystic breast disease and breast cancer; diseases of the ovaries, including polycystic ovarian disease and ovarian cancer; thyroid cancer; prostate cancer; and immune dysfunction, just to mention a few. The RDA for iodine is set ridiculously low at an amount that is insufficient to saturate tissues like the breasts, thyroid and ovaries. A dosage of between 12.5 to 50 mg per day is usually sufficient to normalize iodine levels and to keep levels stable. Dosing may be as high as one hundred mg per day if supervised by a health care provider who can test iodine levels before and during treatment.

Step 2: Alkalinize

One of the most important things a person can do when ill is to move the body to an alkaline state as a matter of urgency. This is done by testing your urine and saliva pH regularly until you achieve an optimal pH. Blood pH is even more helpful but harder to get done because you would normally need a physician to order it for you. The ideal blood pH is 7.365, according to Robert O. Young, PhD, who has spent the last few decades studying the critical importance of maintaining an ideal acid-alkaline balance in the body in order to

optimize health. He recommends urine pH monitoring as a good second option, especially the first urine of the morning, where the pH should be 7 to 7.2 in healthy or slightly health-compromised individuals. The goal should be a pH of 8 in the urine if the individual is dealing with more serious health problems. You should see where you are on the pH scale and make the proper adjustments necessary to remain higher on the pH scale. Proper diet, exercise, nutrients/supplements, and alkaline water consumption are key components in living in an alkaline state.

The Modified Fast and phase 1 of the Green Life Diet are both used not only because they are focused on the intake of low-glycemic index foods, but because they promote rapid alkalinization of the body, which is critical for the improvement of most health challenges, especially chronic ones. Fresh vegetables, except the starchy ones, like potatoes, tend to be alkalinizing. Fruits lower in glycemic index, like grapefruits, lemons, limes, plums, avocados, and kiwis, are also on the list of alkalinizing foods. Organic is always best when available because pesticides and fungicides are acidifying and affect the vitality rating of foods. So much energy has to be used by the detox pathways in our cells and tissues to detox these poisons that not much is left for other vital functions to be able to work optimally.

A diet high in sugars, starches, and processed grains tends to be very acidifying. In general, when you consume lots of dead foods, like highly processed foods, foods cooked at high temperatures, animal-derived foods, and foods full of man-made chemicals, like artificial sweeteners, food coloring agents, MSG, preservatives, and so on, you are likely to be a lot more acid.

Foods like nuts and seeds, dry beans, and moderate-glycemic index fruits and vegetables have little effect on pH either positive or negative. There are some exceptions in the nut group, like peanuts, cashews, and, to a lesser extent, pistachios and macadamia nuts, and in the bean group, like kidney beans and black-eyed peas, which tend to be more acidifying. In the fruit group, you will find that especially tropical fruits are more acidifying because they are higher in gly-

cemic index. This would include oranges, mangoes, ripe bananas, pineapples, and papayas.

You are also far more likely to be successful in alkalinizing your body if you eat right for your blood type and metabolic type and if you avoid foods that you are sensitive to. Other factors that help in alkalinizing your body include the avoidance of alcoholic beverages, tobacco, prescription drugs, and street drugs. Regular light- to moderate-intensity exercise is also a very helpful element to successful alkalinizing. Extreme exercising, on the other hand, can be acidifying because of all the lactic acid generated in the muscles that do not get broken down properly.

Drinking alkalinized, ionized water is another very helpful tool that can greatly facilitate your ability to overcome severe acidity. There are a number of excellent water ionizers/alkalinizers available on the market today that can generate water with a pH as high as 11 on a scale of 1 to 14, which is very alkaline. I would warn, though, that being overly aggressive initially with the consumption of water that is too alkaline can cause severe detox reactions and make you feel exhausted, irritable, achy all over, depressed, and can even cause severe headaches, gastrointestinal discomfort, diarrhea, and nausea. People who suspect that they might have Lyme disease should be especially careful because this organism makes a very alkaline toxin called ammonium causticum, which can cause a metabolic alkalosis, meaning that the body is alkaline from poisoning by this toxin. These individuals are particularly susceptible to severe detox reactions if they are alkalinized too aggressively, even just with diet.

Always start slow when alkalinizing with ionized water by drinking water no higher than 8 or, at the most, 9 on the pH scale, and then bump it up later to higher levels if your pH is not correcting. Also consider the possibility of compromising conditions like diabetes, kidney disease, liver disease, lymphatic dysfunction, or a significant infection with organisms, like fungus, bacteria, or parasites, if the body just won't alkalinize in spite of all efforts. The deficiency of certain nutrients, like sodium, potassium, magnesium, calcium, zinc, copper, manganese, chromium, molybdenum, and other trace min-

Transform Your Life

erals, also can lead to overacidification, which usually responds well to replacement of these essential elements in the body. Salt (sodium chloride) is especially vital. And no, I don't mean table salt, which is an overprocessed, baked-at-extreme-high-temperatures, bleached, and disease-promoting poison. I am talking about minimally processed sea salt, which is rich in trace minerals like iodine, magnesium, potassium, and so on. The serum component of our blood is rich in sodium chloride. In fact, blood is like ocean water if you take the cells and the proteins out.

Stress reduction is also a critical element to alkalinizing successfully. Negative feelings and emotions, such as guilt, shame, sadness, fear, anger, and resentment, are very acidifying, whereas positive feelings and emotions, such as happiness, excitement, passion, forgiveness, enthusiasm, love, joy, and inner peace, help to alkalinize. Actions like laughter, playfulness, gardening, meditation, prayer, listening to inspirational music, learning, and altruism are all additional great ways to help promote this alkalinizing process.

Step 3: Ensure Adequate Water Intake

Over 70 percent of the human body consists of water, and water is needed for every biochemical process that takes place in the body. It is, therefore, no surprise that the most critical substance necessary for the optimal function of the human body is water. Not just any water will do, as we discussed earlier in the book. There is a large problem with contaminants in our water supply—some of them added on purpose by misguided authorities around the country (especially fluoride). The rest are environmental pollutants, such as heavy metals, solvents, petroleum byproducts, pesticides, herbicides, fungicides, plasticizers, bacteria and parasites, even pharmaceutical drugs that can be very difficult, if not impossible, to remove from our water supply through the use of standard water filtration systems used in most communities.

The water that we consume should be as clean as possible with preferably no chlorine or fluoride. If you live in the average com-

munity in America or abroad and get your water from a centralized water supply, you need to be able to filter your water properly. Even ground water can become contaminated with environmental toxins, depending on where you live, and should be tested from time to time to ensure its purity. Certain toxins, such as chlorine, are rather simple to filter out with a basic carbon filter available in most stores selling household goods. Fluoride and other contaminants require more sophisticated filters for efficient removal.

Filtration Systems and Other Clean Water Options

Very good filtration systems are available in the marketplace that will successfully remove chlorine, fluoride, heavy metals, petroleum byproducts, solvents, and microbes, like bacteria and parasites. However, you want to leave in health-promoting minerals. Visit our Web site, www.quantumhealingtyler.com, for more information on some of the best and affordable water filtration system options currently available.

A second option is reverse osmosis, which is a great way to eliminate almost all toxins, but unfortunately, this also eliminates beneficial minerals that are essential to health.

Distilled water may be the cleanest possible source of water, but unfortunately is also completely devoid of all minerals and is very acidic. Distilled water also tends to deplete the levels of minerals in the body because of its diluting effect and its acidity.

Bottled water is another option but comes with its own set of challenges. This includes contamination with plasticizers that even in tiny amounts can have a disruptive impact on the body. Most companies producing bottled water use municipal water supplies as their source of water and often only filter out the chlorine, leaving other contaminants behind. Most bottled water is also relatively acid in terms of pH. Bottled water may be the most profitable business in America with astronomical profit margins when compared with the cost of the actual water that goes into the product.

Transform Your Life

The amount of water that should be consumed on a daily basis depends on a number of factors. This would include the age and weight of the person, the time of year, the activity levels, and the organ functions, among other things. The typical adult would need to drink at least one to two quarts of water per day, but whatever the amount, it should be enough to ensure that the urine stays either clear or light yellow. If it becomes darker, then the person is probably developing a relative deficit in terms of water intake versus water loss.

Alkaline vs. Acidic Water

The water that you drink or cook with also should be alkaline. Most commercial sources of water, including tap water, bottled water, and distilled water, tend to be acidic, or if you're lucky, neutral (distilled water is always acid). Water treated with reverse osmosis is also usually acidic. Any water from these sources can be treated in order to alkalinize them. For instance, distilled water or water treated with reverse osmosis can have minerals and trace minerals added back into them. Minerals tend to be alkaline in nature, whereas mineral-free water tends to be acidic. There are devices on the market that can alkalinize water directly from your tap water source. These are water ionizers, which are electricity-driven devices that can alkalinize water to a pH as high as 11 in some cases. Some of these are sold through direct sales to the public, and then there are some that are marketed through multilevel marketing strategies. The bottom line is no matter what device you use, it should be accompanied by a very good filtration system. Some of these alkalinizers have a rudimentary filtration system that will filter out chlorine and certain other pollutants, but will not filter out fluoride. When you alkalinize water with fluoride in it, you are ensuring even more efficient influx of that toxin into your tissues and into the cells.

One of the great benefits of alkaline water is that you get better water penetration into cells and tissue through the cell membranes and blood vessel walls. This ensures better hydration of the cells and the intracellular matrix. This is critical for proper and efficient detoxification as well. The ideal pH for water is anywhere from 7.4

to 8. For very healthy individuals, an even higher pH can be beneficial. Those dealing with significant health challenges need to be careful not to over-alkalinize initially. When the body starts detoxing and gets acclimatized to water that is mild to moderately alkaline, the water pH can be adjusted to a higher level of 9 or 10 and eventually even as high as 11.

In summary, taking in enough water is critical to your health. It is essential for every function in your body, including all the organs of elimination (bowel, liver, kidneys, lymphatic, skin, and lungs). It is essential for detoxing of the cells and intracellular matrix. In other words, it is critical in the treatment of practically all illnesses. There are a small handful of conditions where increased water intake may be contraindicated. This is especially true when a disease gets close to its end stage (for example, kidney failure and congestive heart failure).

Water is also critical for energy production. You lose strength even with mild dehydration. Unfortunately, most people are not clued in to their body signals and cannot distinguish between thirst and hunger. They also often attempt to satisfy their thirst in a way that can actually make their dehydration worse. Drinking coffee and caffeine-containing beverages and other soft drinks containing high levels of artificial sweetener, even regular sugar, are prime examples.

Water is also critical for normal memory and for effective weight loss. So don't forget, drink enough water.

Step 4: Exercise

Maybe the hardest job for any health care provider in America or anyone in the business of motivating people to help themselves is to get people to exercise. Through more than one hundred years of absolutely phenomenal technological developments, it is now possible to live your life day to day without ever leaving your home or even your couch or your bed. There is an old saying that if you don't use it, you lose it. And your body doesn't just consist of a brain and other key organs, but muscle, bones, and joints that easily become deconditioned when physical activity is limited.

Unfortunately, for too many of us, a sedentary lifestyle devoid of exercise or, for that matter, significant physical activity is par for the course. This is one more reason why as many as 80 percent of adults twenty-five and older are now classified as overweight and why our children are getting more and more overweight at younger and younger ages. There are a number of factors in our society that contribute to this tendency, including too much television and too much time spent on our computers and other gaming devices. Even our military and law enforcement agencies have had to loosen up their criteria in terms of body weight and fitness levels in order to find enough recruits. This should make all of us quite nervous about the long-term prospects of being able to defend ourselves as a nation if this trend continues.

Like most people have a mental block about eating healthy, most people also have a mental block regarding exercise that has to be overcome in order to regain or maintain our health. One of the most important keys to success at improving your level of physical fitness is to reframe the subject of exercise and create a fresh mental outlook. Following are some other suggestions on how to accomplish this.

1. Find something that you enjoy doing that involves significant amounts of physical activity. This may be gardening for one person and home improvement for another. Some really learn to enjoy chores like sweeping, vacuuming, and cutting grass. Others enjoy swimming or dancing or getting together with others and doing yoga, tai chi, or aerobics in a group. Others enjoy the solitude of an early morning or late night workout at a local health club.

2. Change your frame of mind toward physical activity. See yourself in your mind's eye getting stronger and stronger, fitter and fitter, and healthy as a result of moving and using your body.

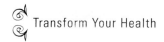

3. Work on identifying and clearing unresolved inner conflicts that are keeping you stuck at home on a couch watching TV instead of out and about, celebrating your magnificent God-given physical body. For example, a conflict regarding lack (i.e., of resources like money) may cause you to become a workaholic, expending all your energy chasing financial wealth and having none left for exercise. Another example is conflict of devaluation (regarding self-image), which may make you too self-conscious to go out in public to exercise, where others might see your so-called imperfect body. There are numerous other conflicts to consider that may have the net result of paralyzing you on this front.

4. Avoid overdoing it when you start an exercise program. So many people make the mistake of violating one of the most basic rules of exercise, which is to start slow and to gradually escalate your intensity over weeks and months. This is essential for avoiding injuries that may put your exercise plans on permanent hold.

5. No excuses. So many people have so many excuses, from lack of time, having too many responsibilities, and being too overwhelmed to having physical ailments that ostensibly limit the ability to exercise. One of the most inspiring stories to me is the story of Christopher Reeve, who never stopped doing whatever he possibly could physically in spite of total paralysis from the neck down after his terrible accident when he was thrown off a horse. He never gave up, until the day he died, on the absolute commitment to getting healed of his paralysis and using his muscles, bones, and joints, even though most of it had to be done with the help of others. He did not do this out of fear of being a quadriplegic for the rest of his life, but because he loved life and loved being able to use his body. He wanted not just to be able to move around, but to be able to show love

and affection to his wife and kids and other friends and family. He was also committed to making an even bigger difference to humanity as a whole.

6. Time your physical activity right to increase the likelihood of long-term success. Researchers have shown that people who work out early in the morning are much more likely to be exercising six months later than those who work out later in the day. The most important reason for this is that you tend to have more energy available to you in the morning, and once you get used to exercising in the morning, it tends to pump you up for the rest of the day, whereas if you wait to work out later in the day, you tend to have less energy and it's more likely to interfere with your sleep habits.

7. Make exercise a priority. If you don't put it in your list of most important things to do, it will tend to slip off your list entirely. This may be one additional reason why working out early is better than working out late.

8. Be accountable. Hold yourself accountable or have someone close to you hold you accountable in a gentle, loving way by reminding you of your priorities and commitments, including your commitment to exercise.

9. Stop procrastinating. Most people have great plans for next week or next month or next year, for instance, when they have more money, more time, fewer responsibilities, and, the worst excuse of all, when they look better and feel more comfortable going out in public. That isn't ever going to happen unless you suck it up and meet your demons head-on. Push through your resistance. Push through your fear, and push through your inertia head-on.

There is so much more to say about exercise, and references are listed in the back of this book to assist you in finding the information and inspiration to take this vital step toward healing.

Step 5: Get Enough Exposure to Sunlight

When it comes to sunlight, our society seems really confused. Instinctively, we seem to know that we need the sun, although most people, especially in the industrialized world, seem to ignore this basic instinct. On the other hand, we have pundits and pontificators that tell us all day long how dangerous the sun is and how high skin cancer rates are soaring because of exposure to the sun, and then peddle their supposedly protective sunscreens and other sun protective products that we buy, spending billions of dollars in the process.

For a greater and greater percentage of our society, protecting ourselves from the sun is a moot point because so many of us seldom even venture outdoors into the sunlight. We live in the shadows with our worlds lit up by artificial light, and we are inundated with indoor pollutants that would normally be destroyed by the sunlight. For thousands of years, entire civilizations have revered and worshiped the sun for its healing properties. Greek philosophers and healers wrote about all the benefits of sunlight. And yet, all of a sudden, here in the twentieth and twenty-first centuries, sunlight exposure is feared, avoided, or heavily protected against. This seems a bit strange, yet there is no arguing that skin cancer rates, including basal cell, squamous cell cancers, and melanoma, are increasing dramatically. It is crazy to believe that sun exposure alone is responsible, seeing that skin cancer rates are rising so rapidly in spite of the fact that we are getting less and less sun exposure on average and are using more and more protection against it. We also are missing out on a ton of great benefits to be gained from regular exposure to the sun.

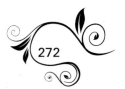

Sunscreens May Be a Double-Edged Sword

One explanation why skin cancer rates are on the increase in spite of the increased use of sunscreens is that ingredients in sunscreen products are causing adverse health effects. Almost all commercially available sunscreen lotions have ingredients that are potentially toxic. The damage from these ingredients includes estrogenic effects, which may promote development of certain cancers, including breast and prostate cancer, some that promote free radical damage to DNA, some that are outright carcinogenic, and so on.

Most sunscreens do not give adequate protection against the most damaging cancer-promoting ultra violet rays of the sun, which are in the UVA spectrum, while protecting against the UVB fraction, which is the fraction critical in the production of vitamin D3 and also most responsible for sunburns. In other words, wearing sunscreens gives us a false sense of security and encourages overexposure to the sun. UVA radiation is present from dawn to dusk, whereas UVB radiation only occurs around the middle of the day. Sunscreens on average also do not protect us as long as advertised, even in ideal circumstances. This is again another reason for a false sense of security when sunscreens are used.

Sunlight and Vitamin D

Hundreds of studies have been done that show that sunlight plays a critical role in healing from dozens of health problems and in the maintenance of health. For example, regular exposure to direct sunlight is essential for the transformation of vitamin D to its active form (vitamin D3), which is a critical nutrient that the majority of us are deficient in these days. Vitamin D deficiency has become almost universal in our society because we don't get enough sun or when we are exposed to sunlight, our skin is unable to make vitamin D3 because of certain things we do. Low vitamin D3 levels may be one of the most common reasons why the cancer epidemic continues unabated. People with high levels of vitamin D are 60 percent less likely to contract cancer overall and, more specifically, cancers like

breast cancer, prostate cancer, lung cancer, and probably even skin cancer. Vitamin D is also critical to bone health for the prevention and treatment of osteoporosis. It is also critical in the prevention and treatment of autoimmune diseases, like inflammatory bowel disease and rheumatoid arthritis; diabetes; heart disease; infections; depression; chronic fatigue; and dozens of other health problems.

Sunlight and Hormonal Cycles

Sunlight is also important in establishing and maintaining normal hormonal cycles, such as the melatonin production cycle by the pineal gland, which increases dramatically during sleep at night if we are exposed to direct sunlight on a regular basis during the day. Melatonin is the body's most important internally produced anti-oxidant and a critical hormone involved in establishing normal sleep rhythms.

The circadian rhythm, which involves the adrenal glands and the cyclical changes in the production of certain adrenal hormones, such as cortisol and hydrocortisone, is also dependent on regular exposure to the sun. Cortisol and hydrocortisone production is supposed to increase dramatically early in the morning—even before we awaken. This plays a critical role in reducing inflammation in the body and increasing energy production in the cells overall. Not enough sunshine, therefore, means not enough energy.

Consequences of Inadequate Sunlight and Benefits From Getting Enough

Not getting enough sunlight also adversely affects the function of your immune system, thereby increasing your vulnerability to infections and even cancer. Not getting enough sun also affects moods and contributes to the rapidly increasing incidence of depression. Getting enough sunlight improves mental awareness, concentration, and productivity, and therefore your ability to learn. Exposure to

sun also improves visual clarity and color perceptions and produces numerous other benefits.

How Much Sun Is Enough?

For the average light-skinned person, twenty minutes of noonday sun is probably enough, and it does not need to be direct sunlight. However, most windows block UV light, which is the most important part of the light spectrum. The eyes need to be exposed to UV light without glasses or contact lenses in order to ensure maximum melatonin production at night. In order to make sufficient vitamin D3, direct skin exposure to sunlight in necessary, with at least 60 percent of your skin exposed to the sun for at least twenty minutes per day. For obvious reasons, if you are very light-skinned, it's probably better to get the sun exposure earlier or later in the day. However, to make vitamin D3 and to reset the pineal gland, the best time to be exposed to sunlight is midday. It is also helpful to use full-spectrum lighting on the insides of our homes and our businesses. Many of the benefits derived from sunlight—like improved mood, awareness, concentration, and productivity; better sleep; and reduced eye strain and fatigue—also are derived from full-spectrum interior lighting when sunlight is hard to come by. Full-spectrum light bulbs are becoming more widely available, although still expensive.

Step 6: Get Enough Fresh Air

Not only do we need sunlight, but fresh air as well. Outside air, even in cities, tends to be much healthier than indoor air, which is filled with indoor pollutants. These indoor pollutants often are concentrated by highly efficient air-conditioning and heating systems, particularly in more energy-efficient homes and businesses. Although these systems do a good job of preventing heat and cold air loss, they also prevent fresher outside air from mixing with dirtier inside air. Inside air tends to be contaminated by outgassing of toxic modern building materials, carpets, paints, and cleaning supplies.

The best option is to spend as much time as you can in nature because not only do you get fresh air and sunlight, but it's great for the soul. Connecting with nature can usually have a phenomenal effect on clearing stress and renewing the spirit. However, it's not possible to avoid indoor air all of the time.

Methods for Improving Indoor Air Quality

There are certain things that can be done to dramatically improve indoor air quality. There are numerous great air filtration systems available from HEPA (high-end particulate) filters to air-ionizing devices that also filter to ultraviolet light systems that sterilize the air of infectious organisms to ozone generators that kill microbes in the air. HEPA filters are very efficient for removing indoor pollutants that involve particulate matter like dust, animal dander, pollen, and fungal spores; however, filters have to be cleaned or replaced regularly. You also get air conditioning unit filters that are HEPA type filters that clean the air in a house much more efficiently than the much cheaper regular filters that most people buy.

Air ionizers work best if they are part of a fan driven filtration system. These devices cause particulate type pollutants to fall out of the air because of the ionizing electrical charges that are transferred to these pollutants. These pollutant particles then fall onto and stick to the elements of the ionizing filter or fall onto solid surfaces where these pollutants can be cleaned off of via other methods such as wiping or vacuuming with a vacuum cleaner. If a vacuum cleaner is used, it too should have a good filtration system. You even get vacuum cleaners these days with HEPA filters in them.

All these measures can be helpful when treating and cleaning indoor air. Ozone, even though helpful for controlling microbes in the air, is irritating to the respiratory tract at higher concentrations and should either be used at low concentrations or when nobody is home and no indoor animals or plants are present. Some companies even combine these different methods of air cleaning into singular devices that can be installed into the duct systems of a central air conditioning unit or can be used as a countertop device.

Plants can make a tremendous difference in improving the quality of indoor air. Full-spectrum light bulbs may help a great deal to keep these plants healthy and strong themselves or otherwise plants can be kept near windows where some sun exposure is likely. It's also important to open doors and windows for long enough periods to allow a home or building's indoor air to be replaced with cleaner outdoor air.

Dust mite excrement and animal dander are two additional large contributors to indoor pollution in many homes. Allergies to dust mite are exceedingly common in our society and often contribute to nasal allergies, chronic sinus inflammation, and asthma. Dust mite allergens can be minimized by covering mattresses and pillows with dust mite covers and treating carpets and curtains for dust mites, or having these removed and replacing them with wood flooring and more rigid window coverings and dressings that can be more easily and thoroughly cleaned. The most allergenic animal dander in domesticated animals is that of cats and allergies to cat dander can also contribute to the conditions listed above especially in those people that own cats. One way to minimize this risk is to clear away cat dander on a regular basis from furniture, bedding, carpets, etc. You can also bathe your cats approximately every two weeks in order to wash off cat saliva, which is the main contributor to cat dander being so allergenic. This practice is obviously fraught with danger seeing that cats hate water. There are cat breeds that have either no dander or less allergenic dander. Unfortunately for some with the worst cat dander allergies, the only option is to find new homes for their cats.

Laptop computers outgas a lot of toxins, including polybrominated diphenyl ether (PBDE), which is a flame retardant, and heavy metals, such as beryllium, mercury, and lead when they are on. Limit use of laptops as much as possible. Use PCs instead. If a laptop is used, use a separate keyboard to increase your distance from the computer itself to minimize exposure to outgassing.

Use green (nontoxic) household cleaning products in your home as much as possible. Standard household cleaning products tend to

be more irritating, allergenic, and toxic than green-rated products. They all contain volatile organic compounds (VOC's) and all standard household cleaners fall under the Hazardous Products Act.

Check for leaks regularly and for signs of mold near water pipes, showers, and so on. Any water leakage in your home that goes undiscovered or unresolved for any length of time will cause mold growth and lead to dramatic increases in mold spores in your indoor air. This will tend to have an adverse impact on the health of those that are exposed.

Avoid the use of commercial fertilizers, pesticides, and herbicides, which may get on shoes and get trampled into your house. These are all made from toxic chemicals that can have devastating adverse effects on health, especially on smaller children and even animals.

Remove shoes before entering your house or at the entrance. This practice helps to reduce the amount of manmade out door chemicals, such as pesticides, fertilizers, herbicides, and fungicides, that are carried into your home contaminating floor surfaces, especially carpets, which are harder to keep clean than hard floor surfaces. Again small children and animals are more vulnerable to these types of pollutants due to contaminated indoor floor surfaces. With that being said, have wall-to-wall carpets removed, especially from bedrooms. This is especially helpful for those who suffer from chronic respiratory illnesses such as asthma, emphysema, and chronic sinus conditions or those that suffer from environmental sensitivity syndrome.

Oxygen Deficiency

We all know what a wonderful thing it is to be able to breathe. This is especially apparent to those who have experienced situations where they were unable to breathe. Those who have choked on something or couldn't catch their breath, like having the wind knocked out of them or sucking water instead of air into their lungs, have a real appreciation for this. Many of us also know how this feels because we may have had a condition like asthma, pneumonia, or severe bronchitis at some point that made it hard to breathe adequately.

Yet, many of us are guilty of improper breathing even when we can. This is because most of us are so busy and under so much stress that we often breathe improperly.

Oxygen is the body's most important nutrient because without it, you can only live for about five minutes. Sufficient oxygen is vital for the optimal functioning of every cell of every organ system in the body and every metabolic pathway in every cell. Cancer, for example, occurs much more readily in organs of the body that receive insufficient oxygen. The same applies to most infections. Most viruses and bacteria are exquisitely sensitive to oxygen and are readily destroyed in the body when oxygen levels are increased to normal in infected tissues inside the body.

It is also important to note that we lose oxygen capacity as we age. It is estimated that the average individual loses about 1 percent of oxygen-carrying capacity per year under normal circumstances after the peak is reached at about twenty-four years of age. This means that 1 percent of our oxygen-carrying capacity that remains is lost each year after age twenty-four.

Breath-saving Measures That Help Us to Heal or Stay Healthy

Focus on deep breathing by doing deep-breathing exercises to increase relaxation and oxygenation. Sounds simple, yet most of us never take the time to do this. When we breathe normally at rest, we use less than 50 percent of our lung capacity, but when we focus on breathing deeply, we use a lot more. Deep breathing for a few minutes every day helps to improve lung function, helps increase oxygen levels in the bloodstream, is very relaxing, and improves mental alertness.

Deep breathing also improves lymph drainage throughout the body by improving lymphatic flow through the lymphatic drainage vessels that come together inside the chest cavity, where they rejoin the blood supply. Most people, especially adults in our society, have poor lymph drainage and don't even know it. One easy way to

check is to look for scalloping of the tongue. Look at the sides of the tongue when you stick it out slightly and when you keep it relaxed while sticking out. Where the tongue presses against the teeth, you will notice little dents if you have problems with lymph drainage. Other signs of poor lymph drainage include swelling of the ankles, tightness in the shoulders and neck, puffiness under the eyes, and stuffiness of the nose, among others.

Here's a deep-breathing exercise for improving lymphatic drainage: Take a slow, deep breath through the nose for the count of seven, filling the lungs to maximum capacity. Hold the breath for twenty-eight counts with the throat kept open, then breathe out very slowly through pursed lips for the count of fourteen, and then repeat. If your lung capacity is smaller than normal, you may use a different ratio; i.e., breathe in on five or six counts, hold for twenty to twenty-four counts, and breathe out on ten to twelve counts. This exercise increases negative pressure in the chest. Holding your breath with your throat open sucks lymph fluid through the lymph vessels into the chest cavity, thereby improving lymph drainage from other areas of the body.

Oxygen supplementation may be very helpful and, in many cases, lifesaving in so many people, especially older adults struggling with chronic health problems. Almost all of my patients fifty-five or over with chronic health problems are studied for signs of hypoxia (low oxygen levels). I have found that the vast majority of them have suboptimal oxygen levels, and a large number have such severe oxygen deficiency at times, especially during sleep, that they would qualify for insurance reimbursement for nocturnal oxygen therapy.

There is great benefit to be gained from optimizing oxygen levels through oxygen supplementation, if necessary. This is particularly important at night during sleep. Optimal oxygen levels are very helpful in treating everything from cancer to heart disease to chronic lung diseases to sleep apnea to chronic infections to a long list of other chronic health problems. Any person suffering from a significant chronic health problem and who is over fifty-five should be evaluated for nocturnal oxygen deficiency and treated with supple-

mental oxygen if they are suboptimal. Athletes know the benefit of oxygen supplementation better than most of us because they know that they recover much more rapidly from fatigue and injuries if oxygen is supplemented in some way. You sometimes see them breathing pure oxygen on the sidelines in between plays in sports like football, and you hear about athletes who own and use hyperbaric oxygen chambers, which help to speed up recovery from injuries.

Step 7: Get Enough Sleep

Sleep deprivation is becoming an ever-increasing problem in our society and affects almost all age groups. Examine your own life, and you will find that you are in all likelihood suffering from this malady as well unless you have been very proactive and live in a pristine environment. Even for those who make every effort to get enough sleep, sleep quality is often suboptimal.

Causes of Sleep Deprivation and Poor Sleep Quality

In our society, there is a growing prevalence of insomnia. This can be associated with the high stress levels that so many of us live with every day. A diet high in sugar; stimulants, like caffeine; and other chemicals, such as artificial sweeteners also contributes to poor sleep quality and poor sleep habits. Vast chunks of our society also have jobs that require them to work at times when they should be sleeping. They then attempt to catch up on sleep during times when good-quality sleep is nearly impossible to come by.

Another big contributor to sleep deprivation is the television set, with its hypnotic effects that mesmerize us into literally spending vast amounts of our lives nailed to a couch, staring at a tube or a plasma screen, vicariously living our lives through others depicted on the TV screen. Most of us have multiple TV sets in our homes so that we can watch TV even in bed. Not only has television become an obsession, but computers and other electronic communication

devices are rapidly catching up, especially when it comes to our youth, where Web surfing, gaming, and endless texting has taken a major foothold. A growing segment of our society lives in relative isolation, communicating with others in little key strokes online or by cell phone.

Adequate High-Quality Sleep and Rest Vital for Health and Healing

For physical healing to take place, in the recovery phase from any illness, it is critical to get adequate sleep. In Recall Healing, the conflict active phase of an illness is signified by the dominance of the sympathetic nervous system, which makes up one of two parts of the autonomic nervous system. Insomnia is prevalent during this phase, and discovering and clearing the underlying disease-causing conflict is critical not only for recovery from the illness, but also to resolve the insomnia. Once the conflict is identified and resolved, the recovery phase kicks in, and insomnia disappears. It is replaced by a period when a lot more sleep is desired and needed in order for the recovery phase to be completed so that the body can be restored to balance. The bottom line is if sleep or rest is inadequate in any way for whatever reason, it makes healing and health maintenance a lot harder, if not impossible, to achieve. It impairs the body's ability to heal itself.

Sleep requirements vary among individuals and by age. Typically from birth to three months old, we need about eighteen hours of sleep and are awake for only six hours daily. This gradually reduces until we are sleeping about twelve to fourteen hours a day by the age of one; ten to twelve hours a day by the age of six; nine to eleven hours a day by the age of twelve; and eight to ten hours a day by the end of our teenage years. It is estimated that the ideal amount of sleep for adults is between seven and nine hours a day. The amount of sleep we need varies a lot, depending on individual variations, environment, stress levels, even the level of consciousness of the individual. When we are functioning at a high level of conscious-

ness or during a period of spiritual high, and at times when we are highly motivated and in maximum creative flow, we tend to need less sleep. When this occurs, sleep needs may decrease sharply for periods of time with no reduction in the level of functioning or in our ability to heal. The reverse is also true, that when we are under siege and operating under high levels of stress, more sleep is usually needed, but harder to come by because of the adverse effects of inner and outer conflicts on sleep quality and sleep length.

Research also has shown that a power nap in the middle of the day has high restorative value on energy and motivation. In some Spanish-speaking countries, it is still part of the culture (the siesta). But as societies become more and more competitive and businesses have to push harder and harder to stay afloat and to thrive, the siesta and even the leisurely lunch are going by the wayside. Certain innovative, cutting-edge companies, however, are reintroducing the siesta to the workplace because studies have shown that a short nap of thirty minutes to an hour's duration dramatically improves productivity and the ability to concentrate among workers.

Other suggestions to ensure adequate amounts of sleep and to improve sleep quality:

1. Make a habit of going to bed at about the same time every night. The best, most rejuvenating sleep is obtained when we go to bed well before 11 p.m., which, according to the organ time cycles, is when the liver and gallbladder go through their optimization cycle.

2. Avoid all stimulants within a few hours of bedtime, including caffeine-containing foods and beverages, foods high in simple sugars, foods containing artificial sweeteners, tobacco products, and so on. Some people are very sensitive to caffeine and either need to avoid it after morning hours or need to avoid it entirely.

3. Avoid food within a couple of hours of bedtime, especially heavy foods, like meat, dairy products, desserts, and other high-sugar, high-fat foods. Alcoholic bever-

ages should be avoided late at night because they also affect sleep quality.

4. Avoid watching television or working on a computer within two hours of going to bed because of stimulation of beta wave activity in the brain, which is associated with increased wakefulness.

5. Do not let your head hit the pillow at night with a head full of unresolved stresses. Write them down in a diary. You may even want to use two diaries—one for positive thoughts to be saved long term, and one for negative thoughts that can be destroyed progressively as you write page by page or in its entirety later on.

6. Do not exercise within four to five hours of going to bed. Exercise increases wakefulness and is best done earlier in the day. Getting adequate exercise, at least three to four hours a week, is very critical for improving sleep quality.

7. Meditation, listening to soothing music, reading, getting a massage, and making love are all good things to do just before bedtime, which may help to improve sleep quality.

8. Slightly sedating herbal teas, like kava kava tea or combination sleep-enhancing herbal teas, or supplements like melatonin, gamma-amino benzoic acid (GABA), 5 hydroxy tryptophan (5 HTP), L-tryptophan, valerian root, magnesium, and vitamin B6 may all be used individually or sometimes in combination to help improve sleep.

9. Avoid tranquilizers and hypnotic drugs as much as possible because of their adverse effects on sleep quality and other side effects even when they are effective in increasing the amount of sleep you get.

Step 8: Reduce Exposure to Foodborne and Environmental Toxins

All processed and artificial foods are filled with unwanted and unhealthy chemicals that have negative effects on health. It seems that no matter how big an effort is made, our attempts to rework foods into anything but the original form or a form very close to it leads to problems. We delude ourselves if we think we can do it better than God. By consuming foods that are heavily processed, we tend to reduce our quality of life in terms of energy and well-being rather than enhancing it. This, of course, is contrary to what the companies that create these products would like us to believe.

One of the key elements of self-healing is effective detoxification, which is very hard, if not impossible, to accomplish when we voluntarily consume significant amounts of highly processed toxin-laden foods. Diet and environmental toxins that need to be eliminated or that can be avoided are discussed in step 10: "Detoxify or Die."

Step 9: Reduce EMF (Electromagnetic Field) Exposure

Very strong electromagnetic fields are produced by all kinds of devices in our modern world. The alarm clock sitting too close to your head while you sleep, the Wi-Fi system radiating your entire house and business, the cell phone or portable phone that you talk on all day long, the local radar weather station, cell phone towers, and satellites all contribute to an ever-increasing dose of EMF radiation that most of us are exposed to on an almost continuous basis. This can have devastating effects on our health. This subject was dealt with in greater detail in an earlier chapter.

More and more people are becoming aware of feeling drained when exposed to high levels of EMF; for example, when they use their cell phones a lot, stand too close to a microwave oven that is in use, sleep with an electric blanket, and so forth. Negative EMF

Transform Your Health

effects on health also can be detected through methods such as electrodermal screening and kinesiology.

The therapeutic approach here obviously is to eliminate or, at a minimum, reduce exposures to high levels of EMF. For example, minimize the use of cell phones and portable phones, use land lines as often as possible, and avoid consuming microwaved foods or getting closer than four feet from a microwave oven that is in use. People who are ill due to EMF may even have to employ a Faraday cage employed over and around their beds to minimize exposure to certain types of electromagnetic radiation during sleep. A Faraday cage is a metal enclosure used to shield individuals from EMF radiation. Wireless devices such as wireless Internet also may have to be eliminated, and some people are so sensitive that they find that they have to move to a location with fewer cell towers in the neighborhood, and away from weather and airport radar systems.

Step 10: Detoxify or Die

In a large part of this book, we have focused on the roots of illness and have emphasized the role of unresolved conflicts as the main cause of illness. We also have reflected on the fact that diseases are biological solutions to these unresolved conflicts, which otherwise would overwhelm consciousness, threatening our short-term survival. So if unresolved conflicts are at the root of all illnesses, what role do toxins play, or, for that matter, infections? We are all aware of the fact that we are facing an ever-increasing amount of man-made toxins and that infections, especially chronic infections, are becoming more and more common. Both of these categories form critical cofactors in disease but are not the main cause of illness.

In an earlier chapter, we discussed the common categories of toxins that we are exposed to and how those toxins contribute to disease formation. In this chapter, the focus is on the cure of illness, which includes the need to reduce the toxic load affecting the function potentially of every organ in our bodies. In discussing the cure, it is critical to note, though, that the load of toxins that we are all

Transform Your Life

exposed to seems to affect each individual differently. Some people develop cancer, others asthma, others even get auto immune diseases, and still others get skin disorders, and so forth. What defines the specific disease that we develop is the specific nature of the unresolved conflicts that we carry within the organ or system that it is downloaded to, with the toxin or infection as the cofactor.

The organ or system that the conflict is downloaded to becomes a toxic focus. For example, an unresolved conflict involving (loss of) territory downloads to the coronary arteries (the heart's blood vessels), and if toxins like mercury from a mouthful of amalgam fillings get into the bloodstream, mercury will accumulate in the coronary arteries. On the other hand, if there is a conflict of separation, the toxic focus might involve the skin. If the conflict is related to not being able to mark one's territory, the toxin will target the bladder. In the rare instance (I have yet to meet such a person) that a person has no unresolved conflicts, the mercury would not settle in any one organ and would readily be excreted from the body.

There is, however, a second consideration, and that is the load of toxin that the body is being exposed to. The larger the load of toxin becomes, the smaller the unresolved conflict necessary to trigger a toxic focus in a specific organ or region of the body.

Mass consciousness also comes into play, whereby a whole community or society or even humanity as a whole may harbor communal unresolved conflicts, leading to an unconsciousness regarding our environment and a greater and greater tendency to pollute the planet and our bodies with impunity. For example, a more materialistic society tends to be far more vulnerable to conflicts of territory; i.e., the threat of losing territory when we are so focused on accumulating possessions. This is the core factor leading to the dramatic increase in the incidence of coronary artery disease that we have seen over the past fifty years or so. When this type of conflict becomes so much more prevalent as it has and intersects with increasing levels of toxicity in our environment and our food supply, it results in a steadily rising incidence of heart disease.

Transform Your Health

Bad Habits

It is undeniable that our habits play a major role in terms of the size of toxic load that we carry in our bodies as well as the types of toxins. For example, if you consume the Standard American Diet (SAD diet), you, in all likelihood, will become very toxic. Again, the types of toxins that we ingest in food were discussed in a previous chapter. Other habits that contribute to toxin accumulation in our bodies include tobacco usage, cleaning our homes with toxic household cleaning products, even certain hobbies can add to our poison load, especially when those hobbies involve noxious chemicals or products that outgas a lot of toxins. Most of our bad habits stem from our false beliefs regarding what is healthy and what is not.

Even our habits in terms of the health care or dental care that we choose have a huge impact in terms of toxicity. Standard conventional care involves the use of drugs, which are almost all man-made and toxic at some level. It is astounding how many people turn a blind eye to the reams of negative side effects mentioned in every ad for drugs on TV and in the media in general. Most people still believe that in spite of the hoard of side effects, including death, prescription drugs are not only the best option, but the only option besides surgery and radiation therapy in the treatment of health problems. This is not only a false belief system, but a very dangerous, potentially life-threatening belief system that when acted upon adds greatly to the toxic load and, by extension, disease promotion in the human body.

The type of dental care that we expose ourselves to also has huge ramifications in terms of our potential exposure to very dangerous toxins. Even though it is widely accepted that mercury is an extremely dangerous toxin, with innumerable studies showing its negative effects on almost every part of the human body, the vast majority of dentists still put mercury right into our mouths without blinking an eye, poisoning patients and themselves in the process. False beliefs regarding the safety of amalgam fillings and the safety of other common procedures, such as root canals, can have devastating effects on health.

It is important to note that even our bad habits affect our health adversely, not just because they lead to increased toxin exposure, but because of their link to unresolved conflicts, including "project purpose" downloads from our parents and other genealogical down- loads. Most of our habits are formed very early in life, and by the age of thirteen, they are pretty much set in stone. We all become programmed on a massive scale not just because of what we have learned from our parents, but also based on the information that we are exposed to at school and especially through the media. Even our government, politicians, medical organizations, insurance com- panies, and the media are complicit in spreading lies about what is healthy and what is not. Blind obedience to authority has been drilled into the vast majority of us. As a matter of fact, we have been wounded into believing falsehoods and have been indoctrinated against listening to our bodies, spirit, and intuition. A majority of humans carry a conflict deserving health. Whether through politi- cal, religious, or social indoctrination, we have been trained to frame ourselves as guilty of innumerable sins and, therefore, have to hope and plead for forgiveness from our Creator or His intermediaries or our fellow human beings. We also feel like we have to place ourselves at the mercy of a paternalistic health care system that often treats us like children who can't think for ourselves and who need to be told what to do and punished with disapproval and sometimes even be ostracized if we don't follow the treatment regimens prescribed by those empowered by the system.

Again, it is appropriate to remind you that in the context of toxicity, the body was created in extraordinary and miraculous ways to protect and heal itself. Now, we must get out of the way. In spite of the monstrous abuse that our bodies take at the hands of our bad habits and false belief systems, our bodies truck on and survive for an average of over eighty years. Effective detox, therefore, requires us first and foremost to resolve false beliefs by fostering an open mind, by educating ourselves, and by not following the party line. We must show courage and determination in the face of adversity and ridicule. Secondly, we need to do our best to discover our unre-

solved conflicts and downloads that form the root not just of illness in general, but also the personality traits, bad habits, and fractured relationships that contribute to our tendency to poison ourselves. Thirdly, we need to remember that we have mechanisms within our bodies that make every effort to protect us against the invasion of toxicity into our bodies and to clear this toxicity if our external defense mechanisms fail to contain toxicity before it spreads to our tissues and organs.

Reduce Exposure

I would like to be able to say that we can avoid exposure to toxins, but in today's world, unfortunately, this is a bit of a pipe dream. Our earth is being deluged by literally thousands of man-made chemicals. In the United States alone, there are over 80,000 chemicals registered for use with a couple of thousand more being added every year. Even unborn fetuses are not exempt from exposure. In one study, umbilical cord blood samples showed contamination with an average of 180 carcinogenic chemicals and an additional 107 contaminants that may contribute to ill health. In addition, over 80,000 metric tons of carcinogenic chemicals are spewed into our air annually in the United States alone. In countries like China and India, statistics are not available, but all indications are that it is far worse, with a lot of those chemicals causing global contamination. In spite of the best efforts to clean municipal water supplies, over 2,000 chemical pollutants are still found on average. These include pollutants such as drugs, pesticides, petrochemical pollutants, and even parasites and bacteria. What is even worse are toxic chemicals added to water on purpose, like chlorine and fluoride, supposedly to keep us from getting sick, but instead contributing dramatically to our toxic load.

In addition, tons of really unhealthy disease-promoting chemicals are added to our food supply and consumed by the vast majority of our population on a daily basis. Add to that a plethora of toxic household chemicals, poisonous additives to skin and hair care products, and toxic lawn care and pest control products, and you can see

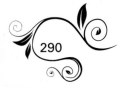

why we are becoming more and more toxic every day. Fortunately, there are steps you can take to reduce your exposure.

Basic Steps to Reducing Exposure to Toxins

1. Eat organic foods, especially fruits and vegetables, as much as possible. Attempt to ensure that all of the foods you eat, grains, meats, and dairy included, are organic. More and more grocery and health food stores are making these available, especially in the bigger cities around the United States, Canada, most of Europe, Australia, and New Zealand. Even though organic products tend to be more expensive than their toxic counterparts, market forces are steadily bringing prices down. If organic is unaffordable to you, consider growing your own. With greenhouse technologies as advanced as they are and becoming more affordable, you can do this year-round in most parts of the world today.

2. Drink plenty of purified spring water, but make sure that both chlorine and fluoride are filtered out, and do your best to avoid water in standard plastic containers when you can. Not only do most plastic containers leach chemicals into water, but the plastic containers themselves have become huge pollution hazards on our planet. If water is not your favorite beverage, there are plenty of other healthy liquids that you can enjoy, including organic herbal teas and freshly juiced fruits and vegetables. A limited amount of organic coffee (no more than one to two cups a day) can be a healthy addition to your daily beverage consumption. Nonorganic coffee is estimated to have one of the highest concentrations of pesticides by weight compared to any other food.

3. Limit your exposure to air pollutants. The ideal is to

Transform Your Health

live in cities or areas with less air pollution. However, most people are not in the position where they can just move to a new location. With indoor air containing on average five times the amount of air pollutants as outside air, spending as much time as you can outside is helpful. Indoor pollution can be markedly reduced with air-cleaning units that ionize and filter air at the same time. Low levels of ozone also can be helpful to sterilize indoor air without irritating or harming airways of people or their pets.

4. Eliminate toxic household chemicals and replace them with products that are less noxious and irritating. These are easy to find in more and more health food stores or on the Internet. Also use barrier devices, such as gloves, when you have to work with toxic chemicals.

5. Use toxin-free personal care products, including skin-cleaning and conditioning products, makeup, and hair-care products. Consider eliminating poisonous hair dyes and nail products by learning to appreciate your natural beauty without them. There are natural hair dyes available that do not poison the scalp or the body. These are available in health food stores and on the Internet.

Support the Body's Detox Organs

Just as the body was built to efficiently digest, absorb, and assimilate nutrients, so was it built to efficiently excrete waste products, including toxins. In the previous section, we discussed ways to reduce our exposure to toxins. It is just as critical to help our bodies be more efficient at excreting toxins. In this section, we are going to discuss various ways in which to support the body to be successful in accomplishing this mission. Our bodies were wondrously created to withstand this withering onslaught of toxicity, allowing for an aver-

age lifespan of eighty-plus years in most industrialized countries. It is conservatively estimated, though, that the average life expectancy even without wondrous new anti-aging strategies should be closer to 120 years or more if we can learn to better take care of ourselves.

Basic Steps to Improve Detoxification

Step 1: Limit Average Daily Calorie Intake

Research on a wide variety of animal species from rats and mice to primates has consistently shown that average life expectancy increases anywhere from 30 percent to as much as 50 percent when calorie intake is reduced. It seems that the increase of maximum life expectancy is achieved by reducing calorie intake about 30 percent below normal satiety levels. In other words, in these experiments, they first established how many calories an animal would eat when there is no limit to the food that is available to it. It was then fed an amount that was, on average, 30 percent less than this amount.

One of the main reasons that this seems to happen is because of the dramatic reduction in the amount of toxic byproducts produced in the body when calorie intake is reduced, especially when those foods consumed are less calorie-dense and have a high vitality rating; e.g., fresh organic vegetables and fruits. When the intake is largely made up of high-calorie-density foods with low vitality ratings—i.e., animal products, processed grains, and refined sugars—there is an increase in the amount of toxic byproducts, and calorie intake is much harder to control. It is easy to overeat on these foods, whereas it is nearly impossible to overeat when the largest percentage of food consumed consists of low-calorie-density foods that are high in vitality rating. Healthier foods, such as fresh vegetables and fruits, especially organically grown, not only reduce the toxic load, but also provide the energy, enzymes, and antioxidants to support and optimize the function of our detox organs.

Step 2: Increase the Intake of Foods Low in Calorie Density That Are High in Vitality Ratings

Eliminate highly processed toxin-laden foods, and reduce (or eliminate) animal proteins. This is the only feasible long-term mechanism by which lower calorie intake can be achieved without a chronic sense of deprivation, which almost always leads to failure. This has been proven repeatedly in studies on obesity, where the average failure rate to maintain weight loss averages 95 percent over two years and 98 percent over five years.

Step 3: Optimize Bowel Function

There are a series of steps that are necessary to ensure that toxins are successfully eliminated from the body. The most critical of these steps is to ensure that our most critical detox organs are working optimally. Maybe the most critical of these is the intestinal tract. The very same rules that apply to optimal nutrition also apply to optimal detoxification. Good elimination, you can say, starts at the very top. In other words, it is very important to chew food well so that the stomach and small bowel have an easier time digesting and absorbing nutrients, thereby reducing the food source for parasites, fungi, and pathogenic (toxin-producing) bacteria in the large bowel. In the same vein, the stomach has to produce enough stomach acid and enzymes to break down especially proteins, and the pancreas and lining of the first part of the small bowel have to produce enough enzymes for further breakdown of foods.

The next important step is for the lower part of the small bowel to be able to efficiently absorb the optimally broken-down nutrient particles. These steps are also necessary in order for the small bowel to be able to absorb sufficient amounts of high-vitality nutrients to allow all of the body's detox organs to be able to function optimally. It is necessary in many instances to support the function of the stomach and the small bowel by adding acid-forming supplements, such as betaine hydrochloride (turns into hydrochloric acid in the stomach) and digestive enzymes, to meals until these organ func-

tions normalize. Many individuals also need certain special nutrients to assist in the repair of the lining of the upper intestinal tract. These may include nutrients such as L-glutamine or herbs such as licorice root or aloe vera.

The next step is to support the growth of health-promoting microbes in the intestinal tract. The average human intestinal tract contains about six pounds of microorganisms. In a healthy individual, these organisms live in a symbiotic relationship with the host, producing essential nutrients necessary for optimal health and assisting in the breakdown of food particles that cannot be absorbed. Dysbiosis occurs when a significant percentage of the organisms in the intestinal tract are toxin-forming and destructive. This condition adds to the load of toxins that have to be eliminated by the liver and the kidneys. Besides improving digestion and absorption and the quality of foods consumed, it is also very helpful in many instances to take a good probiotic. Probiotics consist either of health-promoting bacteria, such as acidophilus or lactobacillus, or sometimes even health-promoting fungi, such as saccaromyces. All of these organisms produce natural antibiotics that suppress the growth of disease-promoting organisms.

Healthy elimination is the next critical step in optimal bowel function. It is critical to eliminate often and thoroughly, which means having at least two to three bowel movements a day. It is normal when optimally healthy to have a bowel movement within thirty minutes to an hour of consuming a meal. This involves a neurological reflex that is suppressed in a large percentage of the population. There are many reasons for this, including the fact that most people don't listen to their bodies due to social customs and end up losing or at least suppressing this reflex. Another reason is the inadequate intake of fiber. In order to promote healthy elimination, it is critical to get enough soluble and insoluble fiber intake. A healthy diet consisting of large amounts of vegetables and fruits typically provides plenty of fiber. Healthy true whole grains can be added unless there is a contraindication to the intake of grains initially; i.e., in people with chronic fungal infections such as chronic candidiasis.

Another key to optimal elimination is the intake of plenty of purified water. This was discussed in greater detail in a previous section.

Step 4: Optimize Liver Function

The liver is an extraordinary organ that is responsible for the elimination of the largest amount of toxins in the human body by far compared with any other detox organ, including the kidneys. Everything discussed so far in this section, including the optimizing of bowel function and the reduced intake of unnecessary food-borne toxins, is critical to help the liver to function at its best. Liver detoxification is generally divided into two phases: phase 1 and phase 2. It is critical for these two phases to be working equally well; otherwise, toxin load can actually increase. For instance, if phase 1 is working well, but phase 2 is not, this can result in certain toxins becoming even more poisonous and can therefore do more harm. This happens, for example, when you consume alcohol. With a small amount of alcohol, it is easy for the liver to metabolize it with minimal buildup of the toxin aldehyde, which results from phase 1 detox and is much more poisonous than alcohol itself. If phase 2 works adequately, aldehyde is rapidly metabolized to nontoxic metabolites.

Phase 1 liver detoxification requires oxygen. Toxins like pharmaceuticals, alcohol, street drugs, and fungal toxins are oxidized in special components of cells called mitochondria, the energy generators of the cells, to make them more water-soluble. An enzyme system called the cytochrome P450 system forms the most important part of phase 1 detoxification in these mitochondria, and many drugs detoxified through this system often interact with one another, causing potentially serious or even fatal harm. This detoxification process routinely generates free radicals, which play a primary role in the development of degenerative diseases and in aging itself. These free radicals may damage the mitochondria themselves, thereby compromising the production of energy.

In order to protect cells from these free radicals, the body uses circulating chemicals called antioxidants and protective enzymes

Transform Your Life

that are part of the phase 2 liver detoxification system. This system is responsible for the complexing of oxidized chemicals with nutrients such as sulfur, specific amino acids, or other compounds in order to efficiently excrete these chemicals in the bile or urine. The antioxidants that are used for disarming free radical chemicals are mostly derived from food or manufactured in our cells. The body needs a full complement of antioxidants such as vitamin A, vitamin C, vitamin E, lipoic acid, coenzyme A, coenzyme Q10, carotenoids, bioflavonoids, and minerals, such as magnesium, chromium, copper, manganese, selenium, molybdenum, sulfur, and zinc.

The healthiest way to obtain these antioxidants is through a very healthy diet containing large amounts of fresh organic vegetables and fruits. Most people either do not have access to sufficient quantities of these foods or choose not to eat this way. Taking antioxidants in supplement form may help to some degree and may even be essential if the body is severely depleted of antioxidant stores. However, one big mistake that a lot of people make is to consume one or two antioxidants—i.e., vitamin E and vitamin C—while neglecting the rest. This may actually be more harmful than not taking any antioxidants at all. For example, one study done on smokers in Finland showed that taking large doses of beta carotenoids alone actually increased the risk of lung cancer.

Top Dietary Sources of Antioxidants

Vegetables

All colors of vegetables, including green, orange, red, yellow, and purple.
Broccoli
Carrots
Collards
Purple corn
Cabbage
Red cabbage
Bell peppers
Dandelion greens
Kale
Mustard greens
Purple onions
Dulse
Hijiki
Kelp
Nori
Wakame
Spinach
Sweet potatoes
Swiss chard
Pumpkin
Radishes
Tomatoes
Beets
Winter squash

Fruits

Apricots
Black cherries
Blackberries
Blueberries
Cranberries
Cantaloupes
Red grapes
Papayas
Raspberries
Strawberries
Honeydew melons
Apples
Acai
Pomegranates
Noni
Wolfberries

Uncooked Nuts and Seeds

Almonds
Brazil nuts
Hazelnuts
Pumpkin seeds
Sunflower seeds

Legumes

String beans
Pinto beans
Lima beans
Blackeye peas
Garbanzo beans
Green split peas
Kidney beans
Lentils
Navy bean
Black bean

Whole Grains

Slow cooked steel cut oatmeal
Brown rice
Wild rice
Basmati rice
Sprouted grain breads
Dark whole grain rye bread
Wholegrain spelt bread
Wholegrain barley bread
Wholegrain rice pasta

Spices

Garlic
Ginger
Parsley
Rosemary
Sage
Thyme
Turmeric
Cilantro

Supplements

Vitamin A
Beta carotene and related carotenoids
Vitamin C (non-corn based)
Vitamin E (mixed tocotrienols)
Bioflavonoids (quercitin, pomegranate extract, etc.)
Copper
Manganese
Selenium
Sulfur (N-acetyl cysteine, MSM, etc.)
Coenzyme Q10 or ubiquinol
Lipoic acid (preferably R lipoic acid)
Milk thistle

Phase 2 liver detoxification is very heavily dependent on sulfur-containing amino acids, such as cysteine and methionine. Glutathione, which is a complex of three amino acids (a tripeptide) is a critical component of cell detoxification and is also a very important antioxidant. Vegetables such as the cruciferous family, including cabbage, cauliflower, bok choy, brussel sprouts, and also onions and kale are very high in sulfur-containing amino acids. Phase 2 also depends on another metabolic pathway critical for effective detox, which involves the methylation of toxins.

Step 5: Optimize Kidney and Urinary Tract Functions

The kidneys are extraordinary organs that have the capacity to excrete very large amounts of toxins and at the same time maintain fluid, electrolyte and blood protein balances. Most people take their kidneys for granted and tend to abuse them mercilessly by refusing to drink adequate amounts of water and other healthy forms of fluid, forcing the kidneys to work overtime to keep enough fluids in the body to keep it functioning. The kidneys are further strained by the large influx of toxins into the body that have to be excreted in order to allow cells and organs to continue working. This work is made considerably harder because of our poor diets and inadequate fluid intake.

Indiscriminate use of over-the-counter and prescription medications also puts a tremendous strain on this set of organs and is most likely the biggest reason why the rates of kidney failure are going through the roof. Every day over-the-counter drugs like acetaminophen (i.e., Tylenol) and ibuprofen (i.e., Advil and Motrin) are extremely common causes of silent kidney damage, leading to the failure of this organ system to be able to detox adequately. There is a long list of other prescription drugs used for common everyday health problems that are also to blame. This is all leading to an inexorable increase in the number of people standing in line for renal dialysis and kidney transplants with far too few kidneys available.

Again, it is important not to forget that the failure of the kidneys to be able to adequately excrete toxins is always linked not just

to the toxic load, but also to those unresolved conflicts that program for weakening or shutdown of the kidneys.

A number of herbal remedies can be helpful here, including parsley, juniper berry, cranberry extract or juice and watermelon seed, and many homeopathic combinations formulated to support kidney functions are available through various homeopathic and homotoxicology companies. Adequate fluid intake, especially water, is critical for optimal kidney function

Chelation Therapy is another valuable treatment option that can be used to enhance not only kidney function but may also improve liver function.

Chelation means "the binding up of toxins" like heavy metals by other chemical agents that are then excreted together through the liver and kidneys. Chelation agents are commonly used in conventional as well as natural medicine to enhance the excretion of heavy metals like lead, mercury, and arsenic, to name just a few. Heavy metal toxicity is exceedingly common and has dramatic negative effects on organ functions, including the kidneys. In order to optimize kidney functions, it is essential to remove heavy metals like lead, mercury, cadmium, arsenic, and uranium. Unfortunately, heavy metal toxicity is hardly ever looked for or treated in conventional medicine. In a previous chapter, the common sources of heavy metal toxicity were discussed. The important thing is that heavy metals contribute a great deal to disease formation, and chelation is a very valuable tool in facilitating their removal. Very powerful chelation agents are available over the counter or by prescription.

Common everyday chelators include antioxidants like vitamin C, glutathione, alpha lipoic acid, and coenzyme Q10. Super green foods that are high in chlorophyll also make excellent chelators. Chlorophyll is not absorbed in the bloodstream, but stays in the gut and is then excreted through the bowel. Certain herbs, like cilantro, are very helpful; cilantro specifically for mercury detox. Ethylenediaminetetraacetic acid (EDTA), dimercaptosuccinic acid (DMSA), and 2,3-dimercapto-1-propanesulfonic acid (DMPS) are examples of man-made chelators that have relatively few side effects if used

Transform Your Life

appropriately and are great chelators for heavy metals like lead, mercury, cadmium, uranium, arsenic, and excessive amounts of copper and iron in the system, which can cause great harm. Intravenous chelation therapy with EDTA has been around for over fifty years. It was originally developed to treat lead toxicity, but was soon discovered to have tremendous benefits in the treatment of cardiovascular diseases, especially those caused by hardening of the arteries (atherosclerosis), with some studies showing up to an 85 percent response rate. These studies that number into the thousands are often criticized for not meeting the highest standards of scientific research; however, it is hard to explain away the fact that millions of people around the globe have mitigated their symptoms and signs of cardiovascular disease through chelation therapy.

There would be a huge economic impact if chelation therapy ever became widely available, was covered by insurance, and started being used in conventional medicine by conventional physicians. This is one reason that conventional medicine is not in love with the approach. By the way, it is entirely possible that certain forms of oral chelation may be nearly as effective as the intravenous forms. There are many oral chelation agents available without prescription.

Step 6: Optimize Lymph Drainage

Optimal function of the organs and cells of the body requires a lymph drainage system that is functioning optimally. This is a requirement in order to remove toxins efficiently from our body tissues so that they can be dumped back into the blood circulation. Most people don't even know that they have a lymph drainage system, and even those who have heard of it don't know how critically important a properly functioning lymph drainage system is for achieving optimal health. Blood circulates through the blood vessels until it gets to the capillaries, which release nutrients into the intracellular spaces called the matrix (also called the ground substance). Nutrients enter the cells from here, and the cells excrete toxins and toxic byproducts of metabolism back into the matrix. The lymph drainage system drains fluids filled with toxins from the matrix through lymph vessels and

lymph nodes and dumps them through the main lymph duct near the heart back into the blood circulation.

Numerous obstacles can arise that may slow down or even obstruct this system. These include an inadequate intake of water (dehydration), a sedentary life style, an overload of toxins, stress, surgical scars, and so on. There are numerous methods that can be applied to improve lymph drainage. These include simple steps like drinking adequate amounts of filtered spring water; and doing aerobic exercise, such as walking, riding a bike, dancing, and rowing. Another great tool that combines exercise and lymph drainage involves bouncing on a rebounder (mini trampoline). Dry skin brushing is also very helpful for improving lymph drainage and requires only a very inexpensive dry skin brush to perform. Instructions on how to perform dry skin brushing can be accessed through our Web site: www.quantumhealingtyler.com. Lymphatic massage is another helpful option and is usually performed by a massage therapist trained in lymphatic massage techniques.

There are also numerous mechanical devices available without a prescription that can be very helpful, including the Chi Machine, which is relatively inexpensive and can be used in almost any location in conjunction with an exercise mat. Far infrared sauna is another technology that is becoming more and more popular and enhances lymph drainage, microcirculation, and detoxification. There are also simple breathing exercises that one can learn that enhance lymph drainage through the main lymphatic ducts that join up to the large blood vessels in the chest. Products can be found on my website for purchase.

Clear Other Common Blocks to Detox

There is a long list of additional issues that can impact negatively on the body's ability to detoxify. Many of these can be handled without professional help, but some may require professional assistance. What may be tougher is figuring out which factors are contributing to your particular health issues and the difficulties that your body may be having in terms of detoxification.

As stated repeatedly in this book, *unresolved emotional conflicts* are a key factor, if not *the* key factor, in programming us for illness and blocking our ability to get rid of toxins. Even in conventional medicine, stress is recognized as a critical contributor to health challenges and is estimated to be the primary reason for 80 percent of visits to physicians' offices and emergency rooms. In a very general sense, the most common negative emotions associated with stress are worry and fear as well as anger and resentment, with other negative emotions like guilt and shame as well as unresolved grief coming into play. It is important to get stress under control or resolved in order to be successful with detoxification efforts. This can only be achieved by identifying and resolving the underlying conflicts leading to the experience we call stress.

It is estimated that as much as 20 percent of adults in our society suffer from fatigue severe enough to be labeled chronic fatigue syndrome. A large contributor to this problem is severe *adrenal exhaustion*, which also contributes to weakness of the detoxification systems. Chronic stress takes a tremendous toll on adrenal function, which, in turn, reduces the available energy for detoxification and healing. Herbal remedies such as schizandra berry, astragalus root, rhododendron, ginseng, and wild yam, either alone or in combination, may be very helpful for improving adrenal resilience. Homeopathic remedies, either alone or in combination, also may help a great deal.

Viruses, bacteria, funguses, protozoa, worms, and other infectious organisms can both weaken detoxification systems and contribute to the load of toxins that the body has to clear. Again, it is important to note that it is not bugs that make us sick, but the vulnerable host that becomes ill. You also can say that stress weakens the immune system, creating an environment in the body conducive to microbial invasion.

When Louis Pasteur first discovered microbes in conjunction with disease, he came to the erroneous conclusion that the microbes were the cause of the disease. This conclusion was further bolstered by the apparent efficacy of vaccinations and antibiotics. However,

Pasteur on his deathbed acknowledged that he was wrong and that the cause of illness associated with infectious organisms had far more to do with factors in the body such as weakness of the immune system and damage to tissues and organs than to the organisms themselves. Sadly, hardly anyone took note of Pasteur's deathbed confession, and to this day, organisms still get the blame for causing disease instead of people recognizing that it is the vulnerable host that is to blame.

Through the work of Dr. Hamer, Dr. Sabbah, and many others, we are learning that microbes act only on command, with the brain as the commander. Microbes are summoned to the rescue by the brain to resolve the physical manifestations of previously unresolved conflicts. Microbes, in other words, only act at the resolution of a conflict and are only virulent during the repair phase. Organs can repair themselves, but this process can take an inordinately long time, with impairment of the corresponding organ systems being prolonged. Organisms such as viruses, bacteria, and fungi play a key role in accelerating the repair phase, sometimes so fast that the breakdown products and toxins formed can foul up the detoxification systems and cause such rapid destruction that it puts the life of the host at risk. This is called a healing crisis. The mitigation of a healing crisis can be life-saving because the infection phase itself leads to increased morbidity and even death. This is one area where pharmaceutical drugs can be helpful and even life-saving, with anti-microbials (antibiotics) and anti-inflammatory drugs the two most helpful categories. Herbal and homeopathic remedies as well as high doses of certain nutrients are also commonly used to mitigate the symptoms of a healing crisis.

The severity of the microbial invasion is directly correlated with the level (severity) and the length (duration) of the corresponding conflict. In cases where a conflict is overwhelming and long-lasting, the microbial invasion can be deadly. The important thing is to recognize that microbes, just like illness, are gifts and evolved with us to be of service during the repair phase of conflicts. What is worrisome is that in this day and age, a number of super bugs have developed

because of the overuse of antibiotics or have been developed by man for nefarious purposes as weapons of mass destruction. These organisms still only act on command of the brain and at the resolution of conflict, but are so virulent that they can much more easily maim or kill. For example, in the case of a terrorist attack with a biological weapon like anthrax combined with the inevitable psychological conflict related to a mass fear of death, the result will be massive lung infection and death potentially on a massive scale.

In the chiropractic field, it has been well-known for over a century that *misalignment of the spinal vertebrae* can affect the nerve roots that exit between the vertebrae and thereby affect organ systems, including the detoxification organs associated with the corresponding nerve roots. Misalignment of vertebrae and other joints also contributes to the formation of toxic focuses in parts of the body where toxins and microbes can accumulate because of nervous system dysfunction in these areas. The most common of these misalignments occurs in the sacroiliac joints, lower lumbar spine, hips, mid-thoracic spine, and the first cervical vertebra.

Malocclusions of the teeth (off-bite of the teeth) also can have significant negative impacts on health and can either cause or result from other spinal misalignments, which, in turn, are associated with regional dysfunction of the nervous system. Malocclusions commonly also contribute to stress in the temporomandibular joints (TMJ), with resultant toxin and microbial invasion in and around this area. Professional help may be needed to correct these structural issues.

Allergies, especially food allergies (and sensitivities), can contribute to dysfunction of the intestinal tract, lymphatic system, and even organs such as the gallbladder, liver, and sinuses, where it can contribute to the formation of toxic focuses in these organs. The end result can be further accumulation of toxins and greater difficulty in excretion of toxins. Food sensitivities are discussed in greater detail in a previous chapter.

Certain *nutrients* are critical in supporting cell functions related to detoxification. We have already discussed the role of antioxidants,

such as vitamin C, vitamin E, lipoic acid, and coenzyme Q10 in reducing oxidation stress in the body. There are dozens of other nutrients that are also critical, including minerals like magnesium and chromium; vitamins, such as the B-complex vitamins; and essential fatty acids, like EPA, found in fish oil. A diet rich in organic vegetables and fruits and other healthy foods high in vitality rating is absolutely critical in maintaining and enhancing the body's ability to detoxify efficiently. Healthy nutrition is discussed in greater detail in a previous chapter as well.

For over 5,000 years, the Chinese have been aware that *scars* can block the flow of energy through the body's meridian system. Any scar on the body that crosses over any one of the fourteen meridians running through the body can affect the flow of energy to the cor-responding organ systems, leading to difficulties in the body's ability to detoxify.

When a scar is formed either through surgery or trauma, it also leads to disruption of blood vessels, lymph vessels, and nerves. Scars frequently become sites of toxin accumulations because of this. There is a third way in which scars affect us. Any deeply felt nega-tive emotion associated with unresolved inner conflicts at the time that a wound is incurred or a surgical procedure is performed will be attached to or associated with this scar.

Scars can be treated and cleared via different methods, including with certain topical remedies, such as bentonite clay, certain trace mineral solutions, or certain homeopathic remedies applied to the scar repeatedly for a few days or weeks. Some of these treatments, however, may only temporarily resolve the negative effects of a scar. Another method that often gives permanent relief involves inject-ing the scars with certain remedies, such as procaine combined with vitamin B12 and certain homeopathic combinations.

Geopathic stress is caused by a naturally occurring, scientifically documented force field, also known as the earth energy grid, also known by names such as ley-lines or the Hartmann Grid. Primitive tribes and animals are intuitively aware of this earth energy grid and will avoid spending extended periods of time, for instance, during

sleep, on these lines because of their potentially negative effects on health. Unfortunately, modern man has lost touch with this natural intuition that would otherwise make him aware of issues such as geopathic stress.

Exposure to geopathic fields over extended periods of time will have negative impacts on organs such as the pineal gland with marked reductions in the production of melatonin, maybe the body's most important internally produced antioxidant, and the hypothalamus, the most critical control center of all the of the hormonal systems. Such exposures also are correlated with a dramatic increase in the risk of cancer and may contribute to numerous other diseases, including obesity.

How can geopathic stress be detected? Many people notice that they seem to feel better when away from their home, or when they sleep in a different bed at home than they usually do. Others may notice that they started feeling ill soon after moving into a new house, or they live in a house that just never felt right. They often wake up still feeling tired no matter how long they sleep. There are also devices available, for example, geo-magnetometers, which can measure local magnetic fields; however, they may not be able to detect all types of geographic stress. These ley-lines also can be detected through dowsing, kinesiology, or electrodermal screening. Eliminating geopathic stress is critical for successful detoxification.

Step 11: Heal False Beliefs

In the spirit-mind-body connection, the mind acts as a relay station that modulates the flow of energy and information from the spiritual domain to the physical domain. Earlier, when we looked at the scale of consciousness, we discussed the fact that people operating at lower levels of consciousness have a much harder time healing. Close-mindedness is associated with lower levels of consciousness and leads to obstruction in the flow of spiritual energy and information into the body. Higher levels of consciousness are associated

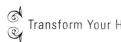

with open-mindedness and a more unfettered flow of energy and information (the spiritual realm to the physical body).

The levels of consciousness in which we operate are correlated with different emotions. At the lower end of the scale, negative emotions and the ego predominate and discernment of truth is nearly impossible so that all of our belief systems are basically those that we have inherited and that we have been indoctrinated with. As we move up the scale of consciousness, we move to more and more positive emotions and have a stronger ability to discern truth. This also is associated with a marked strengthening of our intuition. To know ultimate truth, we need to transcend the ego, our inherited belief systems, and our programmed belief systems.

In the realm of self-healing, it is critical to have an open mind and to strive to operate at the higher levels of consciousness, which also implies that we learn to embrace vulnerability. We have to recognize and eliminate those false beliefs that give most of us a sense of false security in order to allow us to open up to what is true and to get us to where we want to be in terms of optimal health.

The first part of this book focused on the catastrophe happening in health care with an explosion in the incidence of chronic illness, the increased levels of suffering, and despair. This happens in spite of the fact that we are spending absolute fortunes as a society on health care. It seems that the more we spend, the worse things get. When the focus is on symptom treatment and disregards causes, we are operating from a false belief system if we think that that's going to cure anything. However, when we replace that belief system with one that embraces a clear-cut understanding of the root causes of illness, it empowers us immensely along the road of self-healing.

Another false belief system is the belief that toxins and infectious organisms are the root cause of illness. They only interact with and accompany the deeper root cause, which is unresolved conflicts, which have been downloaded into the brain and the body as a survival mechanism. There are tools available to each and every one of us that enable us to discern truth from falsehood, the greatest of which is human intuition. Intuition only comes into play as a consis-

tently available tool when we divorce ourselves from the ego, become humble, and let go of the ultimate stumbling block to growth, which is human righteousness. We are righteous because we are scared to be open-minded and because we are filled with pride. Human righteousness tends to top all other negative emotions and creates a glass ceiling that is hard to break through into higher consciousness.

Another tool that is available to us to discern truth from falsehood is the ability to evaluate the characteristics of our beliefs. Quantum physics teaches us that we are all connected, and the Bible teaches us that God is in everything and everywhere. Belief systems that operate from the concept of separation, selfishness, destruction, and entitlement are more likely to be false, whereas belief systems operating from the concept of oneness and unselfishness are more likely to be true. It also has been shown that when you deeply and profoundly believe in something, whether it is empowering or disempowering, true or false, it is true for you and much more likely to come to flourish. So when you truly believe in miracles, not just for others, but for yourself, then you are much more likely to experience the miraculous. When you truly believe that you can be healed, you are much more likely to achieve healing and better health. When you truly believe that you can be happy and fulfilled, you are much more likely to achieve happiness and fulfillment.

Empowering Beliefs Essential for Healing

The first three empowering beliefs listed here were discussed in a couple of different contexts earlier in this book, but are worth repeating here in the context of empowering beliefs that are essential in order to dramatically increase the likelihood that healing will take place.

1. The belief that you can be healed. If there is even the slightest doubt in your mind regarding the possibility of healing, it will block your ability to heal.

2. The belief that you will be healed. This requires a belief that not only can your disease be healed, but that you will be healed. Again, the slightest doubt will block your healing or lead to reversal over time if healing occurred in the first place.

3. The belief that you deserve to be healed. As many as 60 percent of my patients do not hold this belief at the level of the subconscious when I first start seeing them. They will be unsuccessful because of subconscious guilt leading to a failure to heal, especially long term, unless this belief system is discovered and cleared.

4. A belief in miracles. Most people believe in miracles for others, but often not for themselves. However, when we change our belief systems, we realize that everything is a miracle, including life itself, and we realize that our bodies are constantly healing from second to second and therefore can heal even profound illness if we truly believe that they can.

5. The belief that we are only subject to what we hold in mind. Most of us don't even realize that we create with our very thoughts. Thoughts are things and when strung together over time lead to a reality concordant to our dominant thoughts. When our thoughts shift toward empowerment and wellness, healing becomes far more achievable.

6. A belief that we are infinite beings with an infinite capacity to heal. From a quantum physical perspective, we are infinite in the true sense of the word because our energy field extends from the body into infinity. We are, therefore, more than our bodies and, for that matter, our minds, thoughts, and beliefs. We are spiritual beings having a human experience rather than human beings attempting to have a spiritual experience.

7. Healing is as simple as discovering and clearing the unresolved conflicts that programmed us for our illnesses. We heal by being able to name the illness-causing conflict, claiming it with absolute clarity and dumping it by either resolving the conflict or reframing it.

Step 12: See the Humor in Everything

Laughter is another critical item in your self-healing tool bag. It has been discovered in a group of centenarians that a third key to longevity that they all seem to have in common is a great sense of humor. Those who laugh a lot seem to be a lot healthier in general than those who take life too seriously. Being able to laugh implies the general ability to be able to reframe potentially serious situations in life, to see the humor in them. This was true for Viktor Frankl, who was in prison at Auschwitz Death Camp for over four years and somehow miraculously survived when every other prisoner who had reached prison with him or before him had been put to death. He also survived longer than most of those who arrived after him. Frankl credits his survival to his extraordinary ability to reframe his situation and was even able to find humor in this hellish death camp. Maybe the Germans were so fascinated with him that they decided to keep him alive just to see if his good humor would last, or maybe they were just fascinated by this young man, who refused to give up and who even made a study of his captors to see what made them tick. He would laugh at his co-prisoners when he was successful in manipulating them to give him their vegetables, a few tasteless pieces of throw-away vegetables in the bottom of their soup bowl, in exchange for his bread. He knew he needed vegetables more than he needed bread and was also able to see the humor in it when he grossed out other prisoners and prison guards by catching rats and eating them raw. He was getting essential protein into his system that nobody else got, and he remained relatively healthy while the rest starved to death or were gassed.

 Transform Your Health

Norman Cousins, when he was diagnosed with a terminal illness and told to get his affairs in order, refused all conventional treatment and decided that laughter might be the best medicine. Instead of getting surgery, chemotherapy, and radiation, he went to the local movie rental store and rented every funny movie he could lay his hands on. For months on end, he watched nothing but funny movies for hours each day and healed his so-called terminal cancer.

When you fill your life with laughter, it becomes so much easier to reduce or resolve the unresolved conflicts and biological downloads that sit at the root of all illness. A great sense of humor also is synonymous with a much greater ability to heal. Remember George Burns, the comedian who was still smoking cigars well into his nineties while enjoying great health for his age and still had a sharp enough mind to learn complicated comedy routines? His explanation for his good health, mental acuity, and ability to withstand the toxicity of his lifestyle was his great sense of humor, his passion for life, and his passion for making a difference.

Dr. David Hawkins, in his numerous books on the science of consciousness, repeatedly makes the observation that all the spiritual masters of human history who all operated at the higher end of the scale of consciousness had one thing in common, and that was a great sense of humor. They were lighthearted in their nature. Jesus was noted for His joyful demeanor even in the days and weeks before His crucifixion. Of course, joy and laughter are synonymous.

A number of significant benefits of laughter have been noted in studies done to track its effects on health. Laughter increases pain threshold dramatically because of its association with the release of endorphins in the brain, which act to numb pain and to elevate mood in general. Laughter also stimulates the immune system and increases the release of white blood cells and antibodies to fight everything from infections to cancer. Even with the most serious life-threatening illnesses, it has been shown that laughter makes a huge difference by improving the quality of life and even prolonging life and dramatically enhancing the likelihood of cure.

Many of you may ask how one finds humor, for instance, in a disease like cancer, which is normally framed by most as a horrible disease. The most powerful way to find humor in a disease like cancer is to go through self-discovery and find the unresolved conflicts at the source of the disease. When we get a crystal-clear perspective on these conflicts and are able to name them and claim them, we are then able to dump them by resolving or reframing the conflicts. We also know from the work of physicians like Dr. Ryke Hamer that cancer cure rates may be as high as 92 percent when the conflict that triggered the cancer is cleared and if the conflict of the diagnosis prognosis is avoided or resolved. This means that we absolutely have to avoid taking the diagnosis of cancer too seriously, or if we have, to lighten up. Laughter is the ultimate antidote to taking anything too seriously, including cancer. We also can smile and laugh because our extraordinary bodies with their extraordinary organs are able and willing to act as a repository of these conflicts until we are able to process them and clear them. So instead of being sad and miserable when dealing with health challenges, learn to see the miracle that illness represents and even the humor in it, and laugh yourself back to health.

A merry heart doeth good like medicine: but a broken spirit drieth the bones.

Proverbs 17:22

Keys to Healing With Laughter

1. Learn to laugh at yourself. Most of us take life way too seriously because of the ego always sees itself as threatened and as separate from others, and is always in competition with others for resources, love, status, and so on. When we look at ourselves from a higher consciousness perspective—i.e., through spiritual eyes—we are able to laugh at the illusions and false beliefs that cause us so much misery.

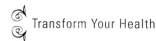

2. Learn to laugh at your imperfections and infirmities. When we realize that we are not our bodies, but that we have a body as temporary housing while we are on this planet, we can laugh at our bodies instead of getting bent out of shape because they aren't shaped perfectly or have lost their youthfulness.

3. Learn to laugh at death. Those of us who have conquered the fear of death tend to live the longest because we are able to live life to the fullest and are able to find joy in every moment. We tend to identify and conquer inner conflicts much more readily, including the conflict relating to the fear of death, which is key to getting and staying healthy. When you are focused on the present and not stuck in the past or in fear of the future, your companion becomes joy, and laughter is synonymous with joy.

4. Learn to laugh at the imperfections of others. When you realize that everyone is divine in essence and yet afflicted with unresolved conflicts stemming from painful experiences of life and related to genealogical downloads from others, it is easy to forgive and have compassion with human imperfections and humans acting out. We are then even able to laugh at our tendency to take things so seriously.

5. Get others to laugh more by encouraging them in a loving way to lighten up. Laughter is the ultimate cure for moodiness and depression and has a phenomenal positive impact on health to the point that it can cure cancer, as Norman Cousins and thousands of others have shown us.

Step 13: Be at Peace with Loss

One of the remarkable statistics of our time is the continuing increase in life expectancy, especially in the industrialized world. In spite of these increases, nobody yet has come up with an antiaging formula that will entirely prevent the demise of our human bodies. The ultimate fountain of youth is yet to be discovered. No matter how much we rail against death and how much we fear it or attempt to avoid it, the fact is that it is part and parcel of the future reality that each one of us has to deal with. Not only do we have to come to peace with our own mortality, but the mortality of those we cherish. In research done on the very oldest among us—i.e., centenarians—certain characteristics stand out about this group. The following pages will deal with these unique characteristics that seem to play a central role in their longevity. Maybe the most important of these is being at peace with loss, seeing that it is such an inherent part of our very existence, whether it's the loss of a loved one, the loss of our own body (death), the loss of function, or the loss of cherished possessions as we age.

Clearing the Conflict Related to the Fear of Loss

Like all unresolved conflicts, the conflict related to the fear of loss needs to be cleared in order to optimize health. We learned earlier that unresolved conflicts can be resolved in one of two ways. Either resolve the problem causing the conflict or learn to reframe it in an empowering way. Since loss is inherent of life itself, resolution in terms of preventing loss is impossible to achieve. That leaves only the second solution, which is to learn to reframe loss in an empowering way.

Realize that We Are All Infinite Beings

In quantum physics, we learn that all material objects, including our bodies, are ultimately made up of pure energy if you break down

matter to its smallest particulates. You also learn that energy cannot be destroyed; it can only be transformed. Another lesson from quantum physics is that consciousness cannot be destroyed and is an inherent characteristic of all that exists, including animate and inanimate objects. This and many other discoveries in quantum physics help us to realize that loss and therefore death of a loved one or our own is no more than an illusion.

Nothing is ever lost in the eyes of God, not a hair on your head, nor a speck of sand.

Overcoming the Conflict Related to the Fear of Death

The Bible and all other religious manuscripts from the world's great religions are full of references to life and the hereafter. Even atheists with a deep understanding of quantum physics understand the concept that consciousness cannot be destroyed. People that make it beyond a hundred are very unique in their ability to continue on and even thrive in spite of the loss of loved ones or possessions or body functions or youthfulness. If you get very old by definition you are going to lose a number of loved ones, including parents, siblings, friends, colleagues, and even members of the younger generation, like children, especially if you make it all the way to three digits.

Staying Connected through Love and Appreciation

Another key characteristic of those blessed with longevity is that they avoid isolation, connect, and make friends easily with others, including those of a younger generation. This is an important hedge against the inevitable loss of loved ones because they always feel loved and appreciated, which stems from loving and appreciating others.

The Path of Nonattachment

If you achieve extraordinary longevity, you are guaranteed of losing not only your body, but a lot of other things, including cherished possessions—as a matter of fact, all of them when you pass on. You are also certain to experience deterioration in the level of function of most of your body parts, if not all of them. You are destined to lose every sign of youthfulness and eventually your body as a whole when you die. Yet, people who make it to a ripe old age typically are at peace with these losses, too. They are able to achieve a certain level of nonattachment to earthly things by taking a more spiritual perspective on life and the objects of the world that surround them. This is one huge disincentive against longevity for the vast majority of humanity.

The Attitude of Gratitude

Being at peace with loss is unimaginable to most of humanity. It is not by accident that the very old among us often have a more spiritual perspective on life and are less likely to get upset about the little details, including chronological aging, gradual or sudden loss of function, and the onset of chronic health problems. An attitude of gratitude is another key characteristic of those who live to a very old age. When you learn to be grateful for everything and everyone, even those who leave your side for whatever reason—whether through divorce; relocation; a change in health status, like Alzheimer's, losing the intellectual relationship without losing the person; and ultimately through death—you are far more likely to be able to identify and clear the hidden conflicts that program for disease and premature death.

Knowing that Life Is Indestructible

We all know that our imagination is so powerful, that we can experience something so vividly through our imagination that it becomes nearly impossible to distinguish between reality and imagination.

This includes being able to experience the presence of a loved one in our mind's eye, even if the person is a thousand miles away or not even on this planet anymore, and we can do this at any time or place, even in our dreams. For many, it goes beyond imagination in the sense that they are convinced of the energetic presence of loved ones, even after a loved one has passed. Not only do they feel their presence, but loved ones come to them in vivid dreams and even sometimes in a visible form while awake. Who knows whether this is real or imaginary, but as we have already concluded, it doesn't matter. Either way, it can be just as pleasing and reassuring. It is no wonder that the people who have had such experiences tend to be far more likely to be at peace with the passing of loved ones.

Overcoming the Fear of Death by Experiencing and Surviving Death

Those who have been through near-death experiences tend to have a very different perspective on death than do the rest of us. Not only do they find an extraordinary peace relating to their own mortality and the mortality of others around them, but they experience massive transformations in their lives in other areas as well. This includes a greater sense of peace with all aspects of their lives, a greater ability to love unconditionally, and far more joy on a daily basis. They usually become far less materialistic and find it far easier to live in the moment.

Seeing the Beauty in Everything

People at peace with loss also tend to be able to see the beauty of this world, even in the aging process itself. They frame aging in a very different light than do most by seeing all the positives related to aging instead of the negatives. This includes the accumulation of wisdom and the relinquishment of stifling attachments that serve no more useful purpose. They celebrate their chronological aging and are undisturbed by the changes that inevitably take place in their

Transform Your Life

bodies. They see the loss of function as coincidental and not of primary importance. They are also able to stay young at heart and find it easy to connect with and enjoy the company of members of younger generations, including children and infants. They also have a greater tendency to be animal lovers. They enjoy the companionship of animals and are at peace with the inevitable loss of these companions to old age. They understand and accept that most domestic animals have much shorter life spans than human beings.

Being at peace with loss is critical to healing. This includes being at peace with a body that is ill or functioning at lower levels. When we are at peace with what is, we have much greater power to bring about what we desire, like healing from a disease or better health in general.

Step 14: Live a Purpose Driven Life

In the surveys done on the growing populations of centenarians, the second characteristic that seems to be pretty universal among them is the fact that they all seem to have had a strong sense of purpose throughout their lives. Living a purpose-driven life means living life with a sense of mission and purpose that transcends just attempting to make ends meet or just being focused on surviving the hardships of life. There typically is a sense of purpose in more than one arena; i.e., career, health, fitness, relationships, child rearing, community service, religious devotion, and spiritual growth, just to mention a few. Those who live the longest tend to be the ones who live life with passion and are in touch with their sense of creativity. They are also less likely to retire early, or if they retire from one career, they usually stay heavily involved in hobbies, community service, or money-making enterprises. They are also the ones who stay passionate and excited about learning new things and expanding their horizons.

Living a purpose-driven life is also a vital characteristic that needs to be embraced by those focused on healing themselves or maintaining optimal health. Motivators for healing can be divided into two categories: negative motivators and positive motivators. Those who grace the earth with their presence for a long time tend to be driven primarily by positive motivators. The same applies to those who end up being successful in their efforts to heal from disease.

Negative Motivators for Healing

Negative motivators for working on your health include fear—the fear of death, fear of suffering, fear of loss of control, and even fear of becoming impoverished. This is especially true for the burgeoning population of uninsured and underinsured individuals and families. If you are uninsured and become ill, not only do you incur the considerable expense of conventional medical care, but also the increased likelihood of losing your livelihood if you fail to get better. For a large percentage of our population, there is no safety net to keep them financially sound if they lose their health and, as a result, are unable to make a living. The most valuable asset we possess is our health.

Negative motivators tend to be weak because they are associated with negative emotions, which place a drain on our life force. They also are less likely to hold our attention for very long, seeing as we have a natural tendency to suppress unresolved conflicts, which is what recurrent negative emotions and recurrent fear and anxiety tend to reflect. Chronic or recurrent negative emotions tend to contribute to ill health. So when we focus on negative motivators as inspiration for the work that needs to be done in order to heal we usually end up failing because of the drain that negative emotions place on our internal energy resources.

Negative emotions also lower the frequency of vibration of your energy field and have negative impacts even on your DNA. Gregg Braden, in his book The Divine Matrix, describes an experiment in which it was revealed that DNA structure was dramatically influenced by the feelings of researchers. Each held a vial containing human DNA while experiencing intense emotions. When the researchers felt love, gratitude, and/or appreciation, the DNA responded by unwinding and the length of the DNA molecule

Transform Your Life

increased. When the researchers felt fear, frustration, anger or stress the DNA molecule responded by constricting and shortening.

This experiment demonstrated that emotions literally impact gene expression by making more or fewer genes available for translation depending on the emotions we feel. Your DNA is able to code for the production of healing proteins and enzymes when you are happy, feeling love, joy, peace, forgiveness, passion, excitement, and so forth. On the other hand, when you experience guilt, shame, sadness, apathy, anger, or fear, for example, there is a reduction in the DNA code available for the creation of healing molecules in the body.

Positive Motivators for Healing

Positive motivators for getting healthy have the opposite effect compared with those of negative motivators. Having a very compelling reason for wanting to heal or wanting to get healthy again is critical to the likelihood of success in your healing efforts. For some people, their main purpose for wanting to heal is to help others heal or to inspire others to higher levels of achievement or it may be as simple as wanting to live life to the fullest and to explore and enjoy their world. There are also those who are motivated by their desire to learn and to better themselves. When you stay focused on a strong and clear purpose in your life and have a strongly compelling positive reason for wanting to heal, it dramatically increases the energy available for healing and the likelihood is far greater of achieving better health.

Step 15: Heal Your Relationships

The third key to exceptional longevity is healthy relationships with others. Dozens of studies have shown that our relationships form a critical key to our overall health. For example, people who are married tend to enjoy better overall health and tend to live longer than those who are divorced or single. Longevity increases even more for married people who rate their relationship very highly compared

with those who give their relationship a low rating. Other interesting findings include the fact that people who feel that they are an integral part of a larger community enjoy better health than those who feel isolated. This also has been found to be the case with people who attend church regularly compared with those who do not. There is a spiritual aspect to this trend, but I think it is safe to say that it also has a lot to do with feeling a sense of community. What strengthens this interpretation is the fact that churchgoing seems to benefit people from many different religions. Churchgoing also tends to feed a sense of altruism. When we are focused on contributing to the lives of others and not just focused on ourselves, we tend to feel more fulfilled in general and are healthier as a result.

Starting in the 1960s, a number of fascinating studies were done to show what a huge impact disruption in the social fabric has on our health. For example, what happens to one spouse health wise seems to directly impact the health of the other spouse. In one study done on men over the age of fifty-five, the death rate among those men soared by over 40 percent during the six months following the death of a wife. Another study showed that men and women who become widowed experience a premature death rate two to four times higher than those still married.

In yet another study, men with coronary artery disease were less than half as likely to experience angina if they rated their relationship with their wives as loving and supportive compared with those who felt isolated and unappreciated in their marriages. In Alameda County, California, a study was done looking at death rates from cancer, heart disease and stroke which are the three most common causes of death for both men and women. They found very strong correlations between certain social influences and decreased death rates in all of these categories. The ones who had the strongest correlation with longevity included those with the largest numbers of close friendships, those who were married, those who were church members, and those who were members of community organizations. A number of more recent studies show that the most common cause of death, which is heart disease in both men and women, and

overall death rates increase dramatically in those who live alone and perceive themselves as lacking friendships or family support or the emotional support of others. This also has been found to be true in women with breast cancer.

A number of fascinating studies have demonstrated the tremendous success of group support strategies in patients suffering from chronic illnesses such as metastatic breast cancer and metastatic melanoma. However, the approach of and premise of the support group has been shown to be critical in whether the group support turns out to be beneficial or harmful. At Stanford University, a large group of women with metastatic breast cancer was studied. These women were treated with the same medical strategies, with the only difference being that about half of the group got to join a weekly support group for one year, whereas the other group did not. This particular support group was led by two therapists, one of who had been a breast cancer patient herself. Group members were encouraged to extract personal meaning from their tragedy and to use the experience of their illness to help others. They also were encouraged to verbalize the effects of the disease on their lives and on their loved ones, and to discuss coping mechanisms that helped them deal with their illness, the pain, and the associated side effects of their medical treatments. The bond between these group members became very strong and continued even after the group sessions ended. The women who participated in the support group lived on average almost twice as long (three years) as members of the control group (nineteen months). This effect of group support is far greater than any medical treatment that could be offered. What was not looked at during the study was how these women dealt with their underlying or unresolved conflicts that had programmed them for their illness. But it seems obvious to me that in this very supportive group setting, the women receiving group support were far more likely to have dealt with their disease-triggering conflict than those women who did not receive group support.

The hidden factor that underlies all other factors discussed above is a greater likelihood of finding solutions to conflicts, or being able

to reframe unresolved triggering or programming conflicts, when we find ourselves in supportive social environments. High-quality relationships also have great physiological benefits because they buffer the impact of stress and strain on the body and mind. These relationships lower the levels of chemical stress mediators such as adrenaline and cortisol. The relationships also tend to correlate with greater self-esteem, self-respect and self-confidence which all lead to better health outcomes. In addition, healthy relationships tend to make us feel like we are more effective in our lives and that we are able to bring about more positive outcomes. They also make us feel that we are making a positive contribution to the lives of others with whom we have a relationship. Having a greater sense of empowerment in our relationships is critical for our health.

How to Create Great Relationships: The Observer Effect

Quantum physics teaches us that we have a direct impact on our inner and outer universe by observing it. In other words, the act of observation itself influences everything around us. In Lynne McTaggart's book The Field, there is a summary of the experiments that have unequivocally proven this. What influences the power of our observations more than anything else in terms of the effect that they have on ourselves and others is how we interpret what we observe with our five senses. It is important to realize that we are also able to observe with something that goes beyond our five senses. Some call this our sixth sense, others call it intuition, and yet others call it our spiritual vision. Our five senses are extremely limited in terms of what they are able to observe, and in order to know our universe, we have to go far beyond them.

Interpret Your Reality in an Empowering Way

What is really important here is not necessarily what we see as our reality, but how we interpret it. This, more than anything, defines our

relationships. Again, the roller-coaster analogy teaches us that two people can go through the exact same physical experience of going down a roller coaster, but have two totally different experiences. The same goes for relationships. If we are tortured by our present reality in a relationship we have the ability to reframe that relationship; in other words, to reinterpret it. We can even change the nature of the relationship by observing it from a different angle.

Have Compassion

Compassion is one answer. I believe that there are no inherently evil people in the world, but there are hoards of people who are programmed to act out in dysfunctional, cruel or evil ways. In quantum physics we learn that everything is connected no matter how far across the universe we go. In a metaphysical or spiritual way we can interpret this to mean that we are all one; therefore, when you are dissatisfied or tormented by those you are in a relationship with you may be able to see that something within you that has not been healed is being reflected back to you in that relationship.

Compassion also grows when we realize that what causes us to act out in negative ways on relationships or to interpret our feelings and what we see as negative has almost everything to do with our programming and the programming of others. Every single one of us comes into this world with our genealogical downloads and then adds the programming and triggering conflicts that each of us acquires from the moment of conception. In addition, when we realize that we are attracted to those things in our universe that reflect incompletion or unresolved conflicts within us it becomes easier to have compassion for ourselves and to become more constructive in every one of our relationships. It is very important for us to realize that our relationship challenges have very little to do with the person we are in a relationship with and far more to do with our unresolved conflicts which program us not just for troubled relationships, but also for health challenges.

Resolve Your Inner Conflicts

Just as our physical health challenges are reflections of our unresolved inner conflicts so are our relationship challenges. Our outer universe is always a reflection of our inner universe and this holds true for our relationships. When we have unresolved anger and resentment within we will almost certainly find ourselves surrounded by angry and bitter people. If we have unresolved conflict of abandonment we are drawn to relationships where abandonment will materialize. If we have unresolved territorial conflicts we will tend to be drawn into relationships and business partnerships where more territorial conflicts are likely to occur.

Resolve Your Fears

In relationships our unresolved fears tend to manifest themselves over and over again creating self-fulfilling prophecies. When we fear abandonment and experience abandonment it reinforces the fear drawing more experiences of abandonment. Our emotions become attractor fields, drawing to us experiences that reinforce how we feel in the first place. So when we are miserable we draw more reasons for misery which reinforces it. Along the same vein, if we are joyful we tend to attract more events into our lives to be joyful about. We may not always feel like we can choose the events of our lives, but we most certainly can choose how we interpret events and how we feel about them. Most people are victims of their downloads and unresolved conflicts, both those inherited through their genealogy and those acquired through their lifetimes.

See Your Relationships as Mirrors

Just like with health, our relationships act as mirrors of our inner state of being creating a constant feedback loop and giving us the ability to see where we are in terms of our inner universe. It seems almost masochistic to torture ourselves based on what is being reflected back at us. When you look at it from this perspective being a victim

in a relationship is almost nonsensical and yet the vast majority of human beings play this game of being the victim which corresponds with the game of being the villain. For there to be a victim, there has to be a villain, and taken from the perspective of the individual, villain and victim become one. Being a victim or, for that matter, a villain is simply a choice and not inherent to any situation. There is always a third choice and that is simply to be in the moment and neutral in terms of judging situations, people, and emotions.

Forgive

Forgiveness is the key to happiness. As our compassion grows for ourselves and others, forgiveness becomes easier and easier. When we realize that being a victim is a choice, just as being the villain is, and that we are able to take a third path of being nonjudgmental and compassionate, forgiveness becomes effortless. We realize that the power of the observer gives us the power to choose our experience in our relationships and thereby are able to create a more empowering reality in those relationships that we decide are meaningful to us.

Be Present in Your Life

Most people are caught in an endless cycle of misery because they are living in their past and are not able to live in the now. The reason why they are unable to escape from a past is because their programming is still running the show and they are seemingly unable to escape the program's hold. Another reason is because of our addiction to certain states of being. We are constantly making attempts to recreate those past experiences that gave us pleasure; in other words, those past experiences that were associated with sharp increases in the brain chemicals that we associate with pleasure. These include endorphins, which mimic the effects of morphine in the brain, and other pleasure-giving chemicals that mimic the effects of drugs like Valium and amphetamines (speed). In a morbid sort of way, we even get addicted to negative states of being, such as anger, depression, and anxiety. Studies have actually shown that people will actively

look for reasons to be anxious, depressed or angry even when everything is seemingly going well.

Becoming the observer is the most critical part of the solution to our relationship challenges. It is only when we step away from ourselves that we are able to see how we are recreating our past and feeding our addictions and can escape these vicious cycles. In this way, we can allow or encourage our negative emotions to be transformed into their positive counterparts. For example, anger can now be transformed into compassion. Fear and anxiety can be transformed into positive anticipation, frustration to excitement, apathy to action, pride to humility and sadness to celebration.

Transform Your Thinking

There is no willpower strong enough to consistently change our thoughts. Seeing that our outer and inner universes are reflections of our thoughts we have to find more effective ways than willpower to change those thoughts if we want to experience more empowerment and greater happiness. This is where becoming the observer is so incredibly powerful. In terms of our health it is critical to note that our thoughts and emotions communicate with our DNA, as described previously. Negative ones make our DNA contract whereas positive thoughts and emotions cause the DNA strands to elongate. This exposes more genes to the inside of our cells that code for the building of proteins and enzymes that are able to repair the body in extraordinary ways. So, in other words, our DNA literally hears everything that we are thinking. Not only that, but our thoughts and emotions also directly impact those around us, as has been proven in quantum physics research. Therefore, changing our thoughts and emotions directly impacts our relationships in extraordinary ways. This allows them to transform, sometimes overnight. Just like miracles happen in the realm of our health so can miracles happen in our relationships.

Empowerment Requires Nonattachment

Again, we hit a paradox. The more intensely we believe we want or need something the less likely we are to get it. This applies to relationships just as it does to the rest of our health universe. God always answers our prayers and always gives us more of what we want and more of what we are focused on, even if our words don't match. If you are focused on the brokenness of a relationship but pray for healing of the relationship you will be left wanting. On the other hand, if you focused on the perfection and beauty of the relationship, no matter what the state of the relationship in the eyes of the rest of the world, you will receive more of what is perfect and beautiful. When I talk about nonattachment I am talking about the choice to be blissful and at peace with whatever our present reality is in terms of our relationships or other aspects of our lives. Being nonattached does not mean that we shouldn't love. As a matter of fact, nonattachment dramatically increases the level of love that we can have for all of those to whom we are connected. It also dramatically increases the level of peace and joy that we can have in our relationships. Again, the more love, peace and joy you see in your relationships, the more love, peace and joy you experience in your relationships.

Suspend Your Own Skepticism and Disbelief

We already discussed in previous chapters the importance of overcoming false beliefs. The problem is that most of us don't know which of our beliefs are false and which of them are true because we are not in touch with our intuition, with our higher selves or with God. Almost all of human suffering and the cruelty of humans toward each other revolve around our beliefs including religion and special interests. Even in one-on-one relationships these two areas create our greatest conflicts. In order to be happy in our relationships and in this world as a whole it is critical that we open our minds to the possibility that we may not always be right. Another's perspective may have some validity to it even though it might be diametri-

cally opposed to ours. It is like two people arguing about what they see when looking at the same quarter from opposite angles. One insists that it is heads and the other insisting it is tails. If they were to switch positions they would see how ludicrous it is to be righteous about their perspective being the only truth. Letting go of righteousness is critical to achieving healthy relationships with other human beings, but requires us to relinquish the stranglehold of the ego.

Are Matches Made in Heaven?

Most people think that when it comes to love, matches are made in heaven. However, most people who tie the knot have rude awakenings after the honeymoon wears off. After the initial infatuation wears off they tend to wake up one day to realize that they hardly know the person they just got married to and start seeing each other's imperfections, which stand in stark contrast to the mainly positive qualities they perceived while they were courting each other. Who they used to feel was the love of their life is now seen in a drastically more negative light.

Most romantic relationships that end up in cohabitation or marriage are based on the genealogical and parental downloads and downloads acquired after conception of the two people involved. You could almost say that each one of us has an almost fatalistic attraction to those who reflect that within us that is incomplete or wounded; in other words, our shadow. This is at least a substantial part, if not the bulk, of what draws us to another as far as romance is concerned. The more we come to terms with and heal our shadow aspect, our unresolved inner conflicts, and our pathological genealogical downloads, the more it allows us to transform our inner universe, thereby changing our outer universe of relationships with others.

Childhood Developmental Stages and Emotional Wounds

What happens to us in childhood during the Oedipal Electra phase of development has a critical impact on whom we choose to get romantically involved with and whom we choose to marry. Between the ages of three and seven years old, we all went through what is called the genital phase of development, where the child becomes aware of his or her genitals. This is also called the Oedipal Electra phase (Oedipal for males, Electra for females). All children go through this phase during which they, under normal circumstances, will literally fall in love for a brief period of time with the parent of the opposite sex. They will actively compete for the affections of that parent and even show aggression toward the parent of the same sex and symbolically want to eliminate or clear away that parent that they for this brief period of time see as an adversarial figure. This phase lasts anywhere from several days to several months, and when handled properly and compassionately by both parents and barring any major traumatic events during this phase allows the child to clear the oedipal complex and reenter the oedipal stage with a sense of indifference toward the parent of the opposite sex, sexually speaking.

If children are traumatized during this stage of development, either by the parent toward whom the oedipal phase is directed or the other parent who is symbolically pushed away, it may have particularly detrimental effects on their romantic relationships later in life. This could include members of the opposite sex or the same sex. There are many aspects of the oedipal phase that affect us later in life, including the type of partner or partners that we choose. In many ways, the partner is a transposition of the parent, but someone that we can create a family with and have sexual relationships with.

For example, a father's scolding a daughter or making a careless or cruel comment during this phase when the daughter is attempting to impress her daddy or look pretty for him may lead to the daughter's having a conflict later related to self-image. An example

of this is what happened to one of my female patients who started dealing with obesity in early childhood, at age five or so. She was prancing around in her leotard after coming back home after a ballet class in front of her daddy one day attempting to impress him with her new ballet moves that she had just learned. The dad made an offhand comment, saying, "No dancing elephants allowed in the living room!" Shattered by his thoughtless and cruel remark she burst out crying and ran straight to her bedroom and slammed the door shut behind her, burying her face in her pillow. Her daddy was the love of her life and she so badly wanted to impress him and win his favor. She was not able to tell anyone, even her mother, what had happened and simply had no choice other than to push it into her subconscious. She also stopped doing ballet then and there, but never would tell her mother why she did not want to go anymore.

Later in life, she gained even more weight, progressively becoming more and more obese until she was over 350 pounds. She also entered romantic relationships with a number of men, attempting to please them in any way she could, just to get rejected over and over again. She was married and divorced three times. Later on in consultation with her during a Recall Healing session involving timeline tracking of her obesity problem she found this and other programming and triggering conflicts. However, this was the big wound that set in motion a series of other events that affirmed her conflict of self-image and abandonment. She also discovered that she had a parental download from her mother who also had a major self-image problem and suffered lots of painful rejections by men. Another conflict was inherited from her father relating to a broken relationship with his mother, who programmed him with destructive behavior toward women close to him, including his wife. This led to her subconsciously attracting relationships with men who tended to treat her with disdain once they got into a sexual relationship with her in spite of her doing everything in her power to get their approval.

Another conflict that she discovered was one related to her wanting to act as a wedge between her father and mother who

always fought like cats and dogs. The other conflict was one related to being deprived of optimal nutrition and a conflict of separation from her mother. Both wounds related to her mother's abrupt cessation of breastfeeding her at the age of three months because her mother did not want to be inconvenienced in her social life.

After discovering and claiming her obesity-causing conflicts she was able to dump them by realizing that she didn't need to sequester these unresolved conflicts in her subconscious anymore, even though it was necessary for her survival at the time. She started losing weight almost effortlessly after these revelations and has since then struck up a great relationship with a mature and caring man who worships the ground she walks on.

Modeling Our Parents

A boy tends to model himself after his father in order to have his mother (love object) all to himself. He takes on all of the conscious and unconscious tendencies of the father. If the father is gentle with the mother he will be gentle. If the father is aggressive toward the mother he will be aggressive toward her and later toward his wife.

The same properties apply to a girl (the female child).

If this phase between the male child and mother goes well he will later attempt to find a woman who resembles his mother in some way. If the mother is overcritical toward his father he will seek this characteristic in the woman he partners with.

If communication is cut off with the mother he will end up with a woman who does not want children or he will end up taking the mother's role in raising the child.

If communication is cut off with the father the son cannot identify with his father because in the eyes of the mother the father is good for nothing. This over-develops his communication with his mother. He will seek a woman who communicates well with her children, but his communication will be problematic.

If the communication is defective or poor between the father and the mother the child serves as intermediary between father and

mother and will find a woman as a partner later with whom there will always be conflict and they will need their children to unite them.

If the mother always criticizes the father the son will have difficulty identifying with the father and the masculinity within himself and will, in turn, seek out a more masculine and dominating partner in either a woman *or* a man.

He also may take the opposite track of his father to meet the requirements of his mother and will be at her service. He will later choose a woman who will feel that he is never good enough, no matter what he does.

If the father always criticizes the mother he will see women as worthless and will become hyper-masculine.

If the father is absent the boy will be unable to identify with the father and will find another to serve as his male model, e.g., a grandfather or a stepfather. He will have great difficulty communicating with his future son, and if there is no father at all, marriage will be impossible for him.

If he identifies with a baby sitter in place of his father and she is in the age group of thirteen or fourteen years old and chasing boys, then he will seek a male partner a little younger than himself. (He has identified with chasing younger boys.)

If he identifies with the grandmother, he will have a woman twice his age. If he identifies with a young girl, he will seek a woman younger than he.

If the father is too strict or authoritative, and he communicates poorly with his children, the son will be unable to identify with his father and seek out a male partner.

For female children, all principles apply in reverse order.

Keys to a Healthy Marriage

1. Forgiveness is the key to happiness.
2. Let go of the need for ownership.
3. Let there be spaces in your togetherness.
4. Ask what love would do.

5. Let go of the need to be right.
6. Be impeccable in your communication.
7. Don't take anything personally.
8. Stop making assumptions.
9. Just do your best.
10. Your relationships reflect who you are.

Step 16: Foster an Attitude of Gratitude

Most of our world looks at diseases and illnesses as curses and calamities caused by arbitrary genetic predispositions combined with unavoidable environmental toxicities and lifestyle-related indiscretions that seem nearly impossible for most of us to control or conquer. This seems to be the case even when we know what we are doing is wrong. We tend to see ourselves as victims of a very cruel world where suffering is the rule rather than the exception. Even when we are in good health and are experiencing relative prosperity, most of us anticipate the loss of function, the onset of disease, and the loss of loved ones as we age. As we know by now, negative emotions contribute to the body's becoming ill. In turn, illness itself contributes to the load of negative emotions that we subject ourselves to creating an endless vicious cycle whereby the energetic healing resources are wasted and chronic suffering becomes a fact of life.

Is there a better way to view illness, a more empowering point of view that may not only reduce suffering from the illness, but may actually dramatically improve our chances of healing completely or at least improving dramatically? Fortunately, there is such an attitude that ensures a far greater likelihood of healing and escaping the endless cycle of misery. The way we experience everything in our lives is not dependent on what happens, but on how we frame it. It is the felt experience that counts, not the lived experience. Remember the roller-coaster analogy mentioned in an earlier chapter. Just as in the roller-coaster ride, when you are faced with ill health your experience of it is totally subjective and not inherent to the disease

itself. Even pain can be framed in different ways, depending on the one that it is inflicted upon.

Maybe the most important attitude in healing is the attitude of gratitude. This attitude is so powerful that it can turn what some may see as the greatest curse into the greatest gift. Having a disease or a symptom does not equal being a victim or being miserable or any of the other negative emotions that frequently accompany our afflictions. Earlier, we learned that disease is a blessing, not a curse. It is the brain's best solution to deal with unresolved inner conflicts that would otherwise threaten our immediate survival by overloading the brain circuitry. Diseases are biological solutions to these immediate threats to our short-term survival. When you look at illness from this perspective it is rather easy to have an attitude of gratitude. I dare say that the more deeply you understand this biological principle the more in awe you will become of your extraordinary body, your extraordinary mind and your extraordinary spirit and how they work together to give you the best chance of living for as long as possible.

When you make the choice to be grateful for everything, no matter what happens or has happened, no matter how many times you have been treated unfairly or feel that life has treated you unfairly, no matter how much pain you have had to endure or even how much you have had to suffer financially or in your relationships, you will be on the road to healing. When you see all of this as a gift, and in the beginning this takes hard work and dedication, you start going from survival mode to thriving. Instead of feeling dragged down in the mud your spirit starts soaring and the cells of your body and the organs as a whole respond with enhanced healing capacity. In order to be grateful it helps to accept the fact that your Creator is an all-loving, peaceful and wise God and not a capricious and cruel God out to torture you during or after your physical existence.

A great exercise is to make a list of all the things that you are grateful for, all the people in your life, even those who push your buttons. Start reframing all of your symptoms and illnesses in the same way, and be infinitely grateful to your organs and your tissues

that take up your unresolved conflicts, allowing your brain and mind to operate at a level that gives you a better chance at overall physical survival. Be grateful to your Creator every day for this extraordinary chance at life and the ability to experience this extraordinary and beautiful universe. Thank God every day for your extraordinary body and its extraordinary healing capacity, no matter what your age or what the state of your physical or mental health. Realize that everything is a miracle. Look around you with new eyes and see your health including your body, mind and spirit in a different light.

Behold the miracle of your existence and even of your illnesses, and by doing so, you open yourself up to the possibility of miraculous healing. Most people see miracles as rare and uncontrollable events and consider those experiencing miracles lucky. Those of us blessed with greater wisdom understand that one man's miracle is another man's everyday experience. The attitude of gratitude allows us to be at peace with what is and enhances our ability to manifest health or anything else that we are passionate about through the power of intention.

One final key to being grateful for everything is the ability to forgive. Forgiveness is the key to happiness. When you forgive you are not letting the other person or other party off the hook. You are setting yourself free. Forgiveness is also critical to healing of spirit, mind, and body.

Step 17: Nurture a Direct Relationship with Your Creator

In the chapter discussing the five levels of healing, the highest level of healing was described as level 5, the level of the spirit body. This is the level at which we get to experience our ultimate connection with a higher intelligence—a creative force that makes our very existence possible. This is also the level of deepest connection with our innate capacity to heal beyond the ego and even beyond rational under-

standing for most of us. It is the realm of religion and spirituality, prayer, deep meditation and miracles.

In order to nurture a direct relationship with our Creator, we need to transcend the ego by transcending the focus on linear reality which involves thought processes constantly focusing on separation from our Creator, others, and from our observable universe in general. In many religions there is a tendency to insinuate that we are somehow separate from our Creator until and unless we do certain things. However, this is obviously a mind construct that makes no sense if you really think about it at the deepest level. In the New Testament of the Bible the statement is made that God is in the heavens and in the earth and everything in between. We learn in church that God is the Creator of all that is, that has ever been and all that will ever be. God is omnipotent, omniscient, and omnipresent. So, in other words, in order to connect at the deepest level with our Creator all we have to do is to turn within instead of searching for Him or praying to Him as if He is on the outside. Prayer often has been disregarded as a healing tool by many, but the body of research on the effectiveness of prayer continues to expand, proving unequivocally that prayer works. Larry Dossey has written numerous excellent books on the effectiveness of prayer with ample references to the scientific literature on the subject. Lynne McTaggart, in her book The Intention Experiment, also has a great summary of the research done on prayer that shows unequivocally the extraordinary power of prayer to heal and also points out the methodological flaws in some of the bigger studies that were supposed to show that prayer does not work as a healing tool. Prayer is a very helpful tool in nurturing a direct relationship with our Creator, but is not enough in itself. Even more important is the flip side of prayer, which is meditation. Someone once said that prayer is talking to God and meditation is listening to God. Most of us talk too much and listen too seldom, not just in our relationship with God, but in our relationship with each other.

We have already discussed the principle that behind every illness and symptom there is an unresolved inner conflict operating

in the subconscious. In order to heal, it is essential to discover and resolve the underlying conflicts. The most powerful way to do this is to reconnect with the source of all things. The innate intelligence that resides at your core encompasses all the energetic and biological information necessary to facilitate healing. By stilling the conscious mind it facilitates this reconnection, making it possible to go beyond our false belief systems which are the main obstacles that stand in the way of healing. It also facilitates the flow of healing energy to our organs and our cells, impacting our very DNA, which contains within it the script for healing.

The essential nature of the creative force of this universe is unconditional love, which is the essential force necessary for healing of the spirit, mind and body. This is also the essential nature of the force that connects all things, including us as human beings. As human beings we can become conduits for this healing force in the healing of others. The greatest healers know that healing does not happen because of them, but can happen through them. They become a vehicle, or a pipeline, through which this innate intelligence flows as a force characterized by unconditional love, compassion, and peace. *Heal Thyself* does not mean that you get to take the credit for healing that takes place within you. The credit always goes to the creative force in this universe that gets to work through you when you are in the right frame of mind. It also doesn't mean that you need to do your healing work alone. As a matter of fact, there is great force in numbers. Matthew 18:20 states, "For where two or three are gathered together in my name, there am I in the midst of them," which means that there is phenomenal power in joining with others, especially those operating at a higher conscious level, and those who are conscious of being conduits for healing. When you are connected with your Source you are better able to distinguish between true healers and false healers. True healers are connected to their Source and false healers are connected to their ego.

It is essential for all of us to realize that we are all healers and that in order to be healed, we accept our responsibility to assist others in healing. This doesn't mean that everyone should go into the

healing profession, but through the love and the understanding and the hugs that we give, we become a conduit for healing. Every selfless act and all kindness bestowed on others becomes an instrument for healing. It is also essential to our own healing to give others the opportunity to connect with us and become conduits for healing on our behalf. By being connected with our Source, we are better able to intuit what it is that we need most at the time to facilitate our own healing. Sometimes we need hugs and cuddling, sometimes we need someone to listen as we share information on our underlying conflicts, and sometimes we need a massage or someone to lay hands upon us. At other times, we may need something more like an herb or homeopathic or, on occasion, even a drug, especially when we are in crisis or going through a healing crisis that needs to be mitigated. The more we nurture a direct relationship with our Creator the stronger our intuition will be to help tell us what we need and when we need it. This will greatly help to facilitate our healing.

Step 18: Altruism—In Service of Life and the Living

Altruism means making a difference in the lives of others. Tony Robbins teaches that besides our survival needs, we all have two spiritual needs to fulfill in order to live a fulfilling life and, from my perspective, in order for us to heal. The first is the need to grow. The second is the need to make a difference in the lives of others. In some of the studies on prayer in which prayer was shown to be effective in helping others to heal it was noted that those doing the praying experienced even more improvement in their health than those for whom they were praying. This is a phenomenal discovery, but one that shouldn't surprise us in the least. Intuitively, we know that we feel better about ourselves and about our lives when we are making a difference in the lives of others. A plumber will tell you that a small pipe with low water pressure and little water flowing through it gets clogged up far quicker than a pipe with a large diameter,

greater water pressure and with water moving through it constantly. Altruism acts in a very similar way. When we become conduits for the flow of love and healing energy through us to others the force and flow of that healing energy increase and transform our whole being into a healing conduit. The healing energy flowing through us contributes to the healing of our own spirits, minds and bodies. In order to maximize the flow of healing energy to benefit others (and ourselves), we have to remain humble. A great paradox exists in this universe in that when we attempt to take credit for the healing of others or for making a difference in other people's lives we diminish our capacity to do so. That does not mean that we should have low self-esteem; it means just the opposite. When you are in the flow it is easier to realize the nature of your true essence, which is divinity itself. No matter who you are or where you are located, God is there. The incredible realization is that your essence is divine and that you are a conduit of God's love and peace. It helps you to accept your greatness without arrogance and helps you to act more and more in divine ways with divine results. Jesus said, "He that believeth on me, the works that I do shall he do also; and greater works than these shall he do … And whatsoever ye shall ask in my name, that will I do …" (John 14:12–13). The power of this statement has phenomenal implications for each of us that is working toward self-healing and the healing of others.

Making a difference in the lives of others also is linked to generosity. A number of studies have shown a direct link between greater generosity and better health and also between generosity and greater happiness. Even in the financial world, it is clear that those who share their abundance with others are much more likely to have greater financial blessings. A generous spirit generates a greater tendency for others to be generous back. There is a story of a little boy living in a small town who went to a restaurant for an ice cream sundae. This little boy grew up in a poor family and had to work very, very hard for the little bit of pocket money that he occasionally got. On this day, he had again received a tiny pittance and looked forward to being able to enjoy his favorite dessert. He walked into the restaurant

and sat down at the counter with his dirty clothes and dirty shoes and the little bit of money that he had clutched tightly in his hands. The waitress, who wasn't having a very good day, gruffly walked up to him and asked him, "What do you want?" The little boy replied, "How much do your ice cream sundaes cost?" The waitress replied, "Fifty cents—is that what you want?" "How much is a little cup of vanilla ice cream," the little boy asked with a little disappointment visible on his face, knowing that he had very little money and would not be able to afford the ice cream sundae. She said, "Twenty-five cents—do you want it or not? I don't have time to stand around and quote you the whole menu." The little boy agreed to have the vanilla ice cream, even though he was yearning for that ice cream sundae. He sat there and ate his little cup of ice cream until every speck was gone, stood up, and left. The waitress went by his seat to clean up his cup, but suddenly became overwhelmed with emotions, tears streaming down her cheeks. On the counter, the little boy had left two dimes and five pennies, the exact difference in the amount that he would have needed to buy the ice cream sundae. This little boy had learned from his grandfather to always be courteous and leave a tip when he went to a restaurant. Knowing that he didn't have enough money to buy his favorite dessert and leave a tip he settled for something less and left an indelible imprint on a woman working as a waitress overwhelmed in her life. It transformed her life in an extraordinary way. This little act of kindness led to her changing her mind-set and becoming a giver. All of a sudden, the tips that she was generating in the restaurant multiplied, and soon she was able to upgrade to an even better job.

Touching the hearts of others expands your heart and puts you in the flow, making it so much easier to heal yourself.

A Twelve-week Action Plan to Manifest Your Miracle

In this section, I will be outlining a step-by-step plan that will make a great difference in your quest to optimize your health or turn around a variety of health problems. Even though a great deal can be accomplished without the assistance of a health care professional, I strongly recommend that you seek professional assistance and guidance if you are dealing with potentially serious health challenges, either already diagnosed or suspected. However, taking the lead on the changes that need to be made is your responsibility and is essential for the achievement of success.

And what about miracles? Yes, all healing is miraculous, even the healing we hardly notice; for example, the healing of a cut or the disappearance of a headache. Bigger miracles take a bigger imagination and a bigger effort to clear away the obstacles preventing your body's natural healing response from kicking in and completing the healing process.

Week One

This week take stock of your health and realize that you are ill or, at a minimum, that your health could be better. Your health is your most important possession. On the first day of this first week, buy yourself a journal and start using it immediately. Spend an hour today contemplating your current state of health and write in your journal, noting where you think you are right now in terms of your overall health and where you want to be.

Use this hour to rate your level of functioning in the following key domains: physical, emotional, mental, environmental, relationship, spiritual, and the financial domain. Use a rating scale of one to ten with ten being the best possible level you can envision and one being the worst. If you need an easy resource to accomplish this, you can go to www.quantumhealingtyler.com and pull off the Holistic Health profile.

Write down compelling reasons why the status quo is just not acceptable any longer and the compelling reasons why you want to heal. The more powerful your reasons, the more likely you will be to achieve your goals. Again use your journal to keep track of what is inspiring you and what drives me to want to heal or to improve your health. Achieve all this in the first hour of starting this program on day one.

Set clear-cut goals of what you want to achieve overall with your health and then in each domain just listed. Your goals will be specific and will include timelines. An example would be: "I am forty pounds above my ideal body weight. I have lost fifteen pounds by the end of my twelfth week and am now at a current energy level of five on a scale from one to ten by week twelve."

Write down in your journal each of the twelve weeks with at least one or two pages dedicated to each week. Write down your specific goals for each week starting with week one. For example:

Transform Your Life

1. This week I am figuring out where I find myself in terms of my overall health and in each of the seven key domains.

2. I am going to set my health goals and will write them down.

3. I will schedule a visit within the next seven days with my physician to get a complete physical done.

Studies have shown, for example, in terms of wealth that those people who set clear-cut goals are far more likely to achieve success than those with no or vague goals. Write your goals down in your journal or on a bulletin board.

Keep your bulletin board with your goals on in a location where they can be viewed more than once a day; for instance in your bedroom or in your bathroom.

Set not only health goals, but also goals in the other key domains of your life. This will include your relationship goals, spiritual health goals, work and career goals, financial goals, goals related to emotional and mental health, and even goals related to leisure and relaxation.

Take a workshop, read a book, or do a teleseminar on goal setting. This is offered through the Quantum Healing Institute in Tyler. For information on this, go to my Web site, www.quantum-healingtyler.com.

Be excited about seeing dramatic improvements in your health. Plan to link your goals with powerful positive emotions, such as excitement, joy, passion, and enthusiasm, which is essential in the quest for better health.

Make use of your journal to get and stay in touch with how you want to feel about your health and about everything in your life. Become proactive by envisioning your goals and linking them with powerful positive emotions that you will continue cultivating to help you fulfill your powerful positive intensions.

Decide now who you want to enlist to help me achieve your goals. Write down a list of people that you can depend on to either

join me in your efforts or that will be a good cheerleader when you hit the proverbial wall from time to time. These helpers may include health professionals that have the kind of reputation that will reassure me that they will be solidly on your side in your quest to improve your health.

Depending on your age and health status, you may want to include a health professional capable of doing a complete physical on me. This is especially important if you are a man and age forty-five or older or a woman fifty years or older even if you are in good health. Set up your appointment(s) this first week so you can get this done no later than the second week.

Make your first dietary changes during this week by eliminating processed or artificial foods high in any form of sugar or those foods that contain artificial sweeteners. This would include soft drinks, candy, baked foods such as cookies, pastries, doughnuts, sugary desserts, fruit juices laced with high fructose corn syrup or artificial sweeteners, etc.

Also start increasing your intake of vegetables and fruits as tolerated. If your vegetable intake, for example, has been minimal, start with two or three portions of vegetables per day lightly cooked. Start increasing your water intake to a minimum of twenty-four fluid ounces per day as you eliminate the intake of unhealthy drinks such as soft drinks, fruit juices with any form of extra sugar added or fluids that contain artificial coloring or flavoring agents.

Start drinking clean, filtered water with at least the chlorine removed.

Transform Your Life

Week Two

This week you are going to take massive action starting with the following steps. Create a vision board with your goals on and pictures that represent those goals and will serve as inspiration and reminders of where you want to be in the next ninety days and beyond. Place your vision board in a location where it is easily visible. paste action steps on your vision board. A vision board is a simple yet powerful visualization tool that helps you to turn your health goals and other goals into powerful words and pictures that help to propel you towards manifestation of what it is that you really want to achieve. It consists of a poster or foam board with cut-out pictures, drawings, and/or writing on it that represents what you really want to achieve.

This week you are going to get a complete physical done if you have not had one within the past six months to a year. It will be done by a reputable health professional that you trust will do an in depth evaluation of your current health status and will level with me to help you get a more realistic perspective on where your starting point is.

This overview of your current health status may also include appropriate blood work depending on your age, gender and based on the specific health challenges that you are currently dealing with. A basic work up if you are a fifty-year-old man or woman or older will probably include a chemistry panel, which will help to evaluate your kidney functions, liver functions, electrolytes, blood sugar, and possibly blood calcium levels; a lipid panel to evaluate your cholesterol levels, triglyceride levels, and sub fractions of cholesterol; a complete blood count if there is any reason to be concerned about anemia or the function of the immune system, for example, in case of fatigue, depression, or recurrent infections of any type; prostate specific antigen if you are a man over fifty years old to help screen for prostate cancer; and a urine analysis if you are male or female to screen for kidney problems, bladder infections, and a handful of other conditions.

Additional tests may also be necessary, for example a cardiac

stress test if you are a male forty-five or older or a female fifty or older and are unfit or have not been exercising regularly. Also consider getting your routine screenings for cervical, breast, and colon cancer as well as for osteoporosis done as recommended depending on your age, gender, family history, or health condition.

This week you are going to start figuring out what your food sensitivities are. Dietary changes to make this week include the elimination of foods that are genetically engineered and therefore much more likely to create food sensitivities.

Remove all wheat and wheat-based products.

Remove all corn and corn byproducts.

Remove all soy and soy-based products unless you are sure that it is made from a non-GMO source.

By removing these foods you may notice fewer symptoms like less water retention, less of a bloated feeling, less fatigue, nasal congestion, and brain fog. This will be confirmation that the foods eliminated have been contributing to your symptoms due to food sensitivities. This week reduce the intake of starchy vegetables such as potatoes. Eliminate processed and fried forms of starchy vegetables such as French fries and mashed potatoes. Also increase your water intake to no less than thirty-two ounces per day.

Eliminate all processed foods containing hydrogenated or partially hydrogenated fats including items like chips, most packaged foods containing grains, French fries, and margarines.

Eliminate all baked goods made with flour that contains potassium bromide as a flour conditioner.

Eliminate all alcoholic beverages from your diet and will stay off all forms of alcohol at least for the next eleven weeks.

This week also start exercising if you have been cleared by your health care professional or are in a low risk group as far as the risk of complications from exercise. Start doing a form of exercise that is aerobic in nature, easy to start and easy to do at home or from home and that doesn't require fancy equipment, for example, a walking program. Start with ten to fifteen minutes per day, three days per week. Combine your aerobics program with stretching from day

one, exercise in moderation and give yourself adequate recovery time in between the times that you exercise. Do your best to avoid the excessive build up of lactic acid in your muscles which will cause symptoms such as muscle soreness and stiffness.

Start spending at least five to seven minutes a day meditating. The best time for this is first thing in the morning or in the early evening. For best results, do both. The goal with meditation is to still the busy mind.

There are all kinds of resources available to help you become successful at meditation including books, CDs, DVDs, and even online courses or teleseminars. Quantum tapping and emotional freedom technique (EFT) are two modalities that are very useful in clearing the negative emotions that have held you back. Teleseminars are offered through the Quantum Healing Institute on EFT and Quantum tapping. Go to my Web site, www.quantumhealing-tyler.com, for a list of resources that are available in this regard.

Read up on meditation this week or listen to a CD, an audiobook, or do a teleseminar on this subject. also do a web search to find information on meditation.

Week Three

Start reading more books and articles on natural health and healing and discover the truth about our failed health care system and health care paradigm that is contributing to unprecedented world wide epidemics of chronic disease. Find a book that deals with your particular health problem using natural therapeutic approaches and go onto the internet to do research on what the root causes of your health challenges might be. At the Quantum Healing Institute we have teleseminars on various health challenges that cover both the root causes and the natural as well as essential conventional approaches that are available and potentially helpful to treat your particular health challenge.

If you are taking pharmaceuticals, go on the Internet and do a search on the specific drugs that you are taking. Get the low down on the benefits but also on the possible side effects that you might not hear about from your health care provider or from the drug company that make the drug. Specifically, find out what nutrient levels or what nutrient benefits are diminished by the drug and what you might need to take to reverse this damage that may be caused by the drug.

Stop eating grains or grain derived foods entirely this week if you are dealing with a significant health challenge including any problems with excessive body weight or any health challenge associated with insulin resistance including adult onset diabetes, hypertension, high cholesterol, fatty liver disease, etc. or if you have any disease related to inflammation including any auto immune disease, osteoarthritis, bursitis, etc.

Further increase your intake of fresh or lightly cooked or steamed vegetables to no less than four portions per day and increase fresh fruit consumption to no less than two portions per day.

In order to improve your body's ability to detoxify more efficiently and in order to improve your health, determine your allergies and sensitivities especially to foods identified so you can avoid these foods. (See page 228)

Transform Your Life

In order to improve your health, work on optimizing your bowel functions this week. (See page 294)

Also figure out this week if you don't already know what your blood type is by getting a blood test done.

If you are dealing with a serious or potentially life threatening illness, start the modified fast this week and you will continue this for at least six weeks. You want to be working very closely with a knowledgably health care provider that will be able to support you in figuring out what conventional as well as natural interventions might be necessary to improve outcomes.

Purchase a good juicer if you don't already Own one and start juicing at least once or twice a day if you are dealing with a more serious health problem as part of the modified fast that you are starting this week.

Start taking supplements to enhance your liver, kidney, gastro intestinal, and lymphatic functions. These may include nutrient formulations, herbal remedies, or homeopathic remedies. Go to www.quantumhealing.com for more information on basic detoxification strategies and specific supplements that may be helpful here.

Slowly increase the amount of time that you exercise and slowly increase the level of intensity to ensure that you avoid excessive lactic acid build up in the muscles. Start doing aerobic exercise every other day for fifteen to twenty minutes. Start adding low-level strength training three times a week for ten to fifteen minutes on the days in between your aerobic workouts. Start with lighter weights and work out one group of muscles every other day, for instance, legs on the second day, extensor muscles including the back of the arms, and back muscles on day four and flexor muscles including the front of the arms, shoulders and stomach muscles on day six. In your strength training regimen, initially use lighter sets of dumb bells and your own body weight to provide resistance; i.e. modified push ups, tummy crunches, leg lifts, leg lunges, etc. Also start each exercise session with stretching for at least five minutes and end your session with five more minutes of stretching.

Get an exercise DVD appropriate for your level of fitness and health that will allow you to exercise in your own bedroom or living room. These can be ordered via the Internet or can be purchased at many bookstores, video rental stores, and even grocery stores. Find someone to exercise with you—an exercise buddy. This may be a family member or a friend.

In order to improve your body's ability to detoxify and in order to enhance your body's ability to heal, identify and resolve issues that make it hard for your body to work optimally. Little things like circular metal around parts of your body. Underwire bra straps, wire rim glasses, etc. can all have subtle but yet very significant effects on your health.

Start getting more sun exposure—at least twenty minutes of full sun around noon on at least 60 percent of you body every day. If contraindicated because of medical issues, such as a history of melanoma, or if you live in areas of the world where it is difficult to obtain direct sunlight from above—e.g., during the winter in the northern parts of the United States or in Canada, the Scandinavian countries, and so on—consider taking vitamin D^3 at least 2,000 to 5,000 IU's per day. You may want to consider getting a vitamin D^3 level checked before you start a vitamin D3 supplement.

Read a good book on spiritual health and healing this week, and if you are a person of faith, do prayer work on a daily basis if you are not already doing so, focusing mostly on thanksgiving payers thanking God for all your blessings.

Week Four

Start renting at least one or two funny movies every week and start watching a couple of funny sitcoms on TV every week. Your goal is to bring laughter back into your life on a daily basis. Start keeping daily notes in your journal of those things that made you laugh each day this week. Make a list of at least a hundred things that you are grateful for in your journal. It will include a list of the people that are or have been in your life that have contributed to your growth, including those that have been antagonistic toward you, knowing that your most challenging relationships are often the ones that you have learned the most from and are now choosing to be grateful for. Count your many blessings and include them in this list. Even write down those things that have been hard for you to see as blessings but have seen as adversity. Now choose to look at everything in you life as a blessing, including those things previously framed as curses because they have contributed so much to your growth and to your desire and commitment to heal.

Read up on your ideal blood type diet and start following the dietary recommendations made for your particular blood type. Also further increase your vegetable intake to a minimum of five to six portions of vegetables per day, with at least 70 percent of it being fresh and the other 30 percent cooked in a healthful way, which may include grilling or wok frying with healthy oil like olive oil or coconut oil at relatively low cooking temperatures.

Increase your fresh fruit intake to three to four portions per day and now eat a diet entirely free of grains, simple sugars, and starchy vegetables.

Drink at least forty-eight ounces of filtered or clean ground water every day and eliminate beverages containing caffeine such as coffee. Green tea is still allowed because it contains very small amounts of caffeine. Also increase your consumption of other herbal teas which you count as part of your water intake.

If you have more serious health problems, you should now be in your second week of the Modified Fast.

 Transform Your Health

Continue to increase the amount and intensity of your aerobic and strength training regimen so that you are now doing twenty to twenty-five minutes of aerobic exercise three days per week and fifteen to twenty minutes of strength training another three days per week. Regular stretching should remain a part of every exercise session and continue to be so from now on.

In order to improve your body's ability to detoxify, get your nutrient deficiencies identified so that they can then be resolved either by further improvements in your diet or by also adding certain necessary supplements. (See page 258.)

In order to improve my health, work on optimizing your liver functions this week. (See page 296.)

You should now be meditating (and praying if you are a person of faith) a minimum of once a day for at least ten minutes total.

Also take time this week to do a relationship inventory. Ask yourself: *Where do I find myself in my relationships with those closest to me?* This week focus on your most important relationship. For example, if you are married, ask yourself: *What is the quality of that relationship on a scale from one to ten, ten being phenomenal and one being extremely dysfunctional?* Make a list of what is working for you in this relationship and what is not. Make a commitment to do more to heal and improve this relationship. Ask yourself: *What would it take to get this key relationship closer to a ten on the relationship scale?* Arrange for and have a meeting with this key person in your life to discuss your ideas for what you would like to do or change to make the relationship better.

Read a good book on healing relationships this week.

Week Five

Purchase a book that has a great reputation for being funny and spend at least ten minutes a day reading it in order to bring more laughter into your life.

Educate yourself on what conflicts your health challenges are associated with and endeavor to enhance your awareness of them and to start resolving or reframing of them. Go to www.quantum-healingtyler.com for more information and educational resources such as articles, DVD's, books, teleseminars, and live seminars that are available to assist you in getting educated on this extraordinary new field of medicine.

This week figure out what your metabolic type is and make adjustments to your diet accordingly.

Check your urine pH first thing in the morning after an overnight fast and get more aggressive with your efforts to alkalinize if your urine pH is running under seven by eliminating most foods that are likely to increase acidity, including all refines sugars, artificial sweeteners, grains, all forms of processed foods, animal products such as meat, eggs, and dairy. Attempt to keep your urine pH at eight if you are ill. Avoid fermented foods if your body continues to be to acidic.

Limit or avoid pesticide-laden foods. Switch to organic vegetables and fruits if those are available in your grocery stores.

If you start getting a detoxification related reaction like increased fatigue, achiness, brain fog, or headache, add back some light animal protein, such as the smaller to medium size types of salt water fish for a few days until your body adjusts further to the other foods that are part of the Modified Fast. You should now be drinking a minimum of sixty-four ounces of purified water and herbal teas per day or more if you are overweight or just very large or tall.

Continue to increase the amount of exercise you are doing now to an average of at least thirty minutes per day six days a week for a total of three hours per week.

Get at a minimum twenty to twenty-five minutes of directs sunlight exposure every day this week.

In order to improve your health, work on optimizing your kidney functions this week. (See page 299.)

Start taking steps this week to reduce you and your family's exposure to EMF (electromagnetic field) pollution. Get a device to take a measurement in every room of your home and in your workplace to figure out what the EMF concentrations are. The concentration should be less than one (0.1 or less if you or one of your family members is very ill).

You should now be meditating (and praying if you are a person of faith) a minimum of once a day for at least ten minutes.

Do at least one special thing every day for the person who is most important to you, such your spouse or significant other.

Read a book on alkalinizing your body and review information on the Internet regarding the effects of food-based pesticides on health.

 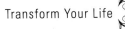

Week Six

If you are having problems following through with the changes that you know you have to make in order to regain control of your health, make the commitment to track down the underlying unresolved conflicts that are at the source of your procrastination and your tendency to self sabotage and that are at the source of your addictive behaviors. Do your best to educate yourself on what these unresolved inner conflicts might be and start doing the work to resolve or reframe them so that you can make better progress toward your goal to be healed.

Continue with the Modified Fast this week and continue to drink at least sixty-four ounces of water per day, even more if you are overweight.

In addition to the formal daily exercise that you are doing six days per week, you should now be looking for additional opportunities to increase your physical activity, including taking the stairs instead of the elevator when you can, walking the dog, parking farther away from the stores where you shop and walking around the mall.

Get at a minimum twenty to twenty-five minutes of directs sunlight exposure every day this week.

In order to optimize your health, work on optimizing your lymph drainage this week. (See page 301.)

Remove cordless phones from your house or place the base in a location far away from bedrooms. Use as seldom as possible and keep the phone on its base as often as possible.

In order to improve your body's ability to detoxify and in order to improve your health, continue to work on discovering and clearing unresolved emotional conflicts programming for disease. (See page 192.)

Get adequate rest. Sufficient and high-quality sleep is a requirement in order to be able to heal. Create an optimal sleep environment by eliminating all light in your bedroom during sleep (low-level red light is okay), minimizing noise, sleep interruptions, and

television watching in the bedroom or elsewhere within two hours of sleep. Avoid eating within two to three hours of going to bed, and before that only eat very light foods, like fruit, fresh vegetables, nuts, or seeds. Avoid any alcohol within two to three hours of bedtime and eliminate caffeine in any form late in the day, depending on how sensitive you are to it. Get at least seven to nine hours of sleep as an adult and more if you are in a younger age group.

You should now be meditating and praying for a minimum of once a day for at least fifteen minutes total.

Read up on the dangers of EMF's by doing an Internet search or by going to www.mercola.com.

Week Seven

Check the pH of you urine first thing every morning and your sputum two or three times per day for five days again to get a baseline on your pH levels. Review the chapter on alkalinizing (See page 262.) to figure out what to do if your pH levels are not responding to the basic dietary changes that you have implemented so far. You can purchase pH paper at certain health food stores, or you can order some through the Web site at www.quantumhealingtyler.com. Continue to check your urine and spit pH once or twice a week until your pH is very consistent at staying within the ideal parameters. At that point you can cut down to once or twice per month on your pH checks or you can stop doing it entirely if you have regained your health and continue to do well.

Continue to follow the Modified Fast; however, if your health has improved and you are feeling a little weak or tired, especially if you are an O blood type, you may want to switch to the Green Life Diet Phase 1 at this point by adding back some light animal protein such as oceanic fish.

Continue to juice at least once or twice a day, using mostly vegetables with a small amount of fruit added in.

Continue to get regular exercise at least six days per week for at least a total of three and a half hours per week.

Get at a minimum twenty to twenty-five minutes of directs sunlight exposure every day this week.

Remove the wireless Internet transmitter (WiFi system) from your home and from your office if possible. Get your Internet hardwired instead.

Continue to work on getting at least seven to nine hours of quality sleep.

You should now be meditating and praying for a minimum of once a day for at least fifteen minutes.

In order to improve your body' ability to detoxify and in order to improve your overall health if you are dealing with significant health problems, you might want to have your hormone levels checked and

get them balanced if necessary. These evaluations might include your adrenals, thyroid, sex hormones, and pituitary hormones such as human growth hormone levels. You may elect to get these treated if they are low, either through natural hormone replacement, homeopathically, or through detoxification and nutrient replacement.

Read a book on natural hormones or do an Internet search on this subject. You can find great books on natural hormone replacement therapy at www.quantumhealingtyler.com.

Week Eight

Start following the Green Life Diet Phase I if you are dealing with a significant health challenge and if you have completed anywhere from two to six weeks of the Modified Fast. This means you can start adding back animal products into your diet. If you started the Modified Fast later than the third week, you may want to continue with it till you get to six weeks total before you switch over.

Eat strictly organic animal products or animal products listed as "free range" such as free range beef, chicken, and eggs. All butter or dairy products that you consume should be labeled as organic, and limit your dairy intake mainly to small amounts of butter—no fat cheese and cottage cheese, low fat yogurt, or kefir with no sugars added.

Continue to exercise at least three and a half hours per week, again focusing on balance. You should now also be looking for more opportunities to play with your kids or grandkids or to play with your spouse or adult friends. Physical play might include kicking or throwing a ball around, playing tag, jumping on a trampoline, swimming, wrestling, tickling, playing charades, etc.

Continue to get at a minimum twenty to twenty-five minutes of direct sunlight exposure every day this week.

Start avoiding the use of microwave ovens entirely, and steer clear of restaurant foods that have been microwaved.

Continue to work on getting at least seven to nine hours of quality sleep.

You should now be meditating and praying for a minimum of once a day for at least fifteen minutes total.

In order to improve you body's ability to detoxify and in order to improve your overall health if you have significant health problems, you should get an evaluation done to discover any significant infections that are affecting your health and to discover any infectious focuses in your body, and then get these treated.

Read up on the dangers of using microwave ovens to cook or heat foods by doing an Internet search on it or by going to www. mercola.com.

Week Nine

If you started on the Modified Fast during week three, it is now time to switch to Phase 1 of the Green Life Diet. Continue to work on alkalinizing your body to within ideal parameters by eating right for your blood type, your metabolic type, based on your food sensitivities that have been eliminated by now, and by focusing on the consumption of a diet that is at least 70 percent alkalinizing foods and 30 percent or less acidifying foods.

Add in some form of exercise associated with a fun activity such as a type of sport, dancing, or yoga in order to avoid getting bored with the same old aerobics, strength training, and stretching every single day. Continue to exercise at least six days per week for a minimum total of three and a half hours.

Continue to get a minimum twenty to twenty-five minutes of direct sunlight exposure every day this week.

Work this week to further reduce your exposure to toxins by eating organic foods as much as possible and by avoiding other unnecessary exposures to toxins, such as mercury in the teeth, immunizations, and common household chemicals. Even most skin and hair care products are full of toxins that are typically not even listed on the label. There is a saying that you should not put anything on your skin that you would not be willing to eat. Go to www.shophealthybody.com for more information on healthy skin care product lines that are toxin-free, and go to any health food store for healthy, toxin-free hair and teeth care products. Avoid products with sodium lauryl sulfate or any other sulfates.

In order to reduce your exposure to EMF's, you should ensure that your alarm clock is more than four feet away from any part of your body.

Continue to work on getting at least seven to nine hours of quality sleep.

You should now be meditating and praying for a minimum of once a day for at least fifteen minutes.

In order to improve your body's ability to detoxify and to improve

Transform Your Life

your health, have your structure (including spine and joints) evaluated and adjusted if necessary.

Read up on the dangers of mercury fillings, immunizations, and toxic skin care and hair care products on the Internet by going to a Web site such as www.mercola.com.

Week Ten

You are now ready to increase the level of intimacy in your relationship with your spouse or significant other, having taken the past six weeks or so to work on that relationship, including daily work on improving communication, forgiving and letting go of the past, and having demonstrated a 100 percent commitment to being the type of person you want your significant other to be in return. Fulfilling the need for love and intimacy is a critical step toward optimizing your ability to heal.

If you started the Modified Fast in week four or earlier, now is the time to switch to Phase 1 of the Green Life Diet or if you started the Modified Fast later and feel drained and tired you may now start adding in some organic animal products that are allowed in Phase 1 of the Green Life Diet.

Continue to exercise at least six days per week for three and a half hours.

Get at a minimum twenty to twenty-five minutes of direct sunlight exposure every day this week.

Get rid of or stop using Bluetooth technologies, especially if you are dealing with significant health problems.

Continue to work on getting at least seven to nine hours of quality sleep.

You should now be meditating and praying for a minimum of once a day for at least twenty minutes.

In order to improve your body's ability to detoxify and heal, have a dental evaluation done to determine and treat significant issues such as having your mercury fillings removed, having root canal teeth evaluated for microcavitations, and to discover and clear malocclusions.

Reminder: If you are having problems following through with the changes that you know you have to make in order to regain control of you health, make the commitment to track down the underlying unresolved conflicts that are at the source of your procrastination and your tendency to self sabotage or that are at the source of your

addictive behaviors. Do your best to educate yourself on what these unresolved inner conflicts might be and to resolve or reframe them so that you can make better progress toward your goal to be healed. Go to my Web site, www.quantumhealingtyler.com, or www.academyCIM.com for a list of resources that are available in this regard. There are educational DVD's available on Recall Healing that can assist you in getting started on figuring out your disease and dysfunction promoting program. Go to www.quantumhealingtyler.com for more information on educational materials such as articles, teleseminars, DVD's, books and live seminars that are available to assist you in getting educated on this extraordinary new field of medicine.

Week Eleven

Continue to increase your consumption of organic fruits and vegetables and depending on your budget and the availability of organic foods, you may choose to start growing your own produce. Go to www.quantumhealingtyler.com for more information on how to get started on growing your own organic produce.

Continue to eat according to the Green Life Diet Phase 1.

Continue to exercise at least six days per week for a total of at least three and a half hours.

Get at a minimum twenty to twenty-five minutes of direct sunlight exposure every day this week.

If you or one of your family members are dealing with significant health problems and if you are living in a downtown or suburban area and are being exposed to very high levels of EMF's due to a high concentration of cell phone towers, start looking into the possibility of moving to a place where exposure will be a lot lower. Also avoid driving or buying a hybrid car.

Continue to work on getting at least seven to nine hours of quality sleep.

You should now be meditating and praying for a minimum of once a day for at least twenty minutes.

In order to improve your body's ability to detoxify, have significant scars checked to see if they are creating interference with any of your energy meridians and get them treated to reverse these effects.

Read a book or look up information on the Internet on the ins and outs of organic gardening and where to find supplies that you will need, including organic seeds, fertilizers, nature friendly pesticides among other things.

Week Twelve

Make a list of the losses that you have suffered through your life, starting from childhood, that you have not been able to come to peace with. This will include the deaths of loved ones, including immediate family, friends, and even pets that you have been unable to transcend emotionally. It will also include losses such as rejection by others through relationship break ups or divorce, job losses, financial or business losses such as bankruptcy, loss of position, etc. Complete your mourning of these losses by using prayer, meditation, journaling, recall healing, or emotional freedom technique, and if this fails, seek psychological counseling. It is critical to learn to reframe and transcend loss in order for healing to take place. Review the chapter in this book on this subject and use your journal to document your victories as well as your struggles in this regard.

Continue onto phase 2 or phase 3 of the Green Life Diet if your health has improved to the point where all symptoms of the health challenges that you started with on day one of your twelve-week plan have disappeared, especially if those health problems are inflammatory in nature or are related to insulin resistance. For example, if you have been successful in getting your body weight down into the ideal range and all other symptoms related to your sluggish metabolism, such as high blood pressure, high cholesterol, high blood sugars, or fatigue have disappeared, then you can move to phase 2 of the Green Life Diet, and if you maintain these improvements for a month or two, you can switch to phase 3. However, you can return to phase 1 if symptoms previously experienced start returning when you switch to phase 2 or 3 or you can continue phase 1 indefinitely and without interruption because it might be easier for you to maintain optimal health on this plan.

Continue to drink at least a liter (close to a quart) of clean, filtered, alkalinized water for every forty pounds of body weight per day unless you physician has instructed you to limit water intake for a medical reason. Make sure the water that you drink is properly

filtered and that all chlorine, fluoride, solvents, and heavy metals are removed.

Get at a minimum twenty to twenty-five minutes of direct sunlight exposure every day this week.

If your health has been restored, you can now drink a small glass of red wine once or twice a week.

Continue doing at least three to four hours of exercise per week balanced between aerobic exercise, strength training, and stretching. Ensure that you are doing forms of exercise that you can enjoy for the years and decades to come and that you continue to look for opportunities to be more active in general.

Continue to work on getting at least seven to nine hours of quality sleep.

You should now be meditating and praying for a minimum of once a day for at least fifteen minutes.

Find out if you are being affected by geopathic stress. Identify and avoid locations prone to geopathic stress.

Read a book on overcoming and transcending loss.

When you have implemented your twelve-week action plan, there is one more thing to do and that is to celebrate! There are many things to celebrate including the improvements in your health that you are bound to have already noticed and many more improvements to look forward to. There is also life to celebrate, love to celebrate, and untold blessings to celebrate. Everything in this incredible universe that we live in is a miracle to behold if we only would open our eyes.

Bibliography

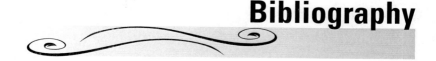

Ballentine, Rudolph, MD. *Radical Healing: Integrating the World's Great Therapeutic Traditions to Create a New Transformative Medicine.* New York: Three Rivers Press, 1999.

Benor, Daniel J., MD. *Spiritual Healing: Scientific Validation of a Healing Revolution.* Volume 1. Southfield, MI: Vision Publications, 2001.

Braden, Gregg. *The Divine Matrix: Bridging Time, Space, Miracles, and Belief.* Carlsbad, CA: Hay House Inc., 2007.

Christiano, Joseph. *Blood Types, Body Types and You.* Lake Mary, FL: Siloam Press, 2000.

Colbert, Don, MD. *Deadly Emotions: Understand the Mind–Body–Spirit Connection That Can Heal or Destroy You.* Nashville: Thomas Nelson, Inc., 2003.

———. *The Seven Pillars of Health.* Lake Mary, FL: Siloam Press, 2007.

Cowden, W. Lee, MD; Ferry Akbar Pour, MD; Russ Dicarlo; and Burton Golberg. *Longevity: An Alternative Medicine Definitive Guide.* Tuburon, CA: Alternative Medicine Books, 2001.

D'Adamo, Dr. Peter J. and Catherine Whitney. *Eat Right 4 Your Type.* New York: J. P. Putnam's Sons, 1996.

Diamond, John, MD. *Your Body Doesn't Lie.* New York: Warner Books, Inc., 1972.

Dossey, Larry, MD. *Reinventing Medicine: Beyond Mind-Body to a New Era of Healing.* New York: HarperCollins Publishers, Inc., 1999.

Dyer, Dr. Wayne W., MD. *Change Your Thoughts—Change Your Life: Living the Wisdom of the Tao.* Hay House Inc. 2007.

————. *Inspiration: Your Ultimate Calling.* Carlsbad, CA: Hay House, Inc., 2006.

Ford, Debbie. *The Secret of the Shadow: The Power of Owning Your Whole Story.* New York: HarperCollins Publishers, Inc., 2002.

Freston, Kathy. *Quantum Wellness: A Practical and Spiritual Guide to Health and Happiness.* New York: Weinstein Books, 2008.

Fromm, Erich. *To Have or to Be? A New Blueprint for Mankind.* London: Abacus, 1976.

Galland, Leo, MD. *The Four Pillars of Healing: How the New Integrated Medicine Can Cure You.* New York: Random House, Inc., 1997.

Hamer, Reiki—Germanic New Medicine Disease Chart.

Hawkins, David R., MD, PhD. *Healing and Recovery.* Sedona, AZ: Veritas Publishing, 2009.

————. *Power vs. Force: The Hidden Determinants of Human Behavior.* Carlsbad, CA: Hay House, Inc., 2002.

————. *Transcending the Levels of Consciousness: The Stairway to Enlightenment.* Sedona, AZ: Veritas Publishing, 2006.

————. *Truth vs. Falsehood: How to Tell the Difference.* Toronto: Axial Publishing Company, 2005.

Hay, Louise L. *You Can Heal Your Life.* Carlsbad, CA: Hay House, Inc., 1999.

Heel Biotherapeutic Index. Authorized by the Medical-Scientific Department of Biologische Heilmittel GmbH, Bade-Baden, Germany. Fifth revised English edition, 2000, p. 9–16.

Hyman, Mark, MD. *Ultra-Metabolism: The Simple Plan for Auto-*

matic Weight Loss. New York: Scribner, 2006.

Miller, William R. and Janet C'de Baca. *Quantum Change: When Epiphanies and Sudden Insights Transform Ordinary Lives.* New York: Guilford Press, 2001.

Obissier, Patrick. *Biogenealogy: Decoding the Psychic Roots of Illness.* Rochester, VT: Healing Arts Press, 2006.

Ornish, Dean, MD. *Love & Survival: 8 Pathways to Intimacy and Health.* New York: HarperCollins Publishers, Inc. 1998.

Padus, Emrika. *The Complete Guide to Your Emotions & Your Health: New Dimensions in Mind/Body Healing.* Emmaus, PA: Rodale Press, Inc., 1986.

Rapp, Doris J., MD. *Our Toxic World: A Wake Up Call.* Buffalo, NY: Environmental Research Foundation, 2004.

Rein, Glen, PhD. and Rollin McCraty, PhD. "Local and Non-Local Effects of Coherent Heart Frequencies on Conformational Changes of DNA." In *Proceedings of the Joint USPA/IAPR Psychotronics Conference.* Milwaukee, WI, 1993.

Renaud, Gilbert, PhD., *Recall Healing: Unlocking the Secrets of Illness.* Self-published by Gilbert Renaud PhD and Recall Healing, Vancouver.

Renaud, Gilbert and Bertrand Lemieux. *Eating Disorders: Obesity, Bulimia, Anorexia and Other Digestive Related Disorders.* Self-published by Gilbert Renaud and Totalbiology Consulting.

Robbins, Anthony. *Get the Edge.* Palm Desert, CA: Guthy-Renker Corp., 2000. Audiobook CD series.

———. *The Time of Your Life.* San Diego: Robbins Research International, Inc., 1998. Audiobook CD series.

———. *Unleash the Power Within.* Niles, IL: Nightingale-Conant Corp., 2005.

Schutzenberger, Anne A. *The Ancestor Syndrome: Transgenerational Psychotherapy and the Hidden Links in the Family Tree.* Hove,

East Sussex: Routledge, 2007.

Sutphen, Dick. *Radical Spirituality: Metaphysical Awareness for a New Century*. Malabo, CA: Valley of the Sun Publishing, 1995.

Trudeau, Kevin. *Natural Cures "They" Don't Want You to Know About*. Elk Grove, IL: Alliance Publishing Group Inc., 2004.

Truman, Karol K. *Feelings Buried Alive Never Die*. St. George, UT: Olympus Distributing, 2003.

Wordsworth, Chloe Faith. *Quantum Change Made Easy: Breakthroughs in Personal Transformation, Self-Healing, and Achieving the Best of Who You Are*. Scottsdale, AZ: Resonance Publishing, 2007.

Wright, Henry W. *A More Excellent Way: Be in Health*. Thomaston, GA: Pleasant Valley Publications, 2005.

Young, Robert O., PhD. and Shelley Redford Young. *The pH Miracle: Balance Your Diet, Reclaim Your Health*. New York: Wellness Central–Hachette Book Group, 2002.

———. *The pH Miracle for Weight Loss: Balance Your Body Chemistry, Achieve Your Ideal Weight*. New York: Wellness Central–Hachette Book Group, 2005.

Resources

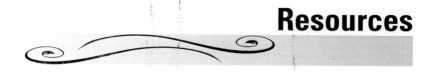

Visit my Web site at www.quantumhealingtyler.com for more information on the subjects covered in this book.

Visit www.shophealthybody.com for access to sources that you might need on your journey back to health.

Contact the Quantum Healing Institute at:
212 Grande Blvd, Suite C114
Tyler, TX 75703
Phone Number: (903) 939–2069

For additional information on the subject of Recall Healing, go to www.academyCIM.com for online courses on Recall Healing taught by Gilbert Renaud, PhD, and David Holt, DO, HMD. Also visit Gilbert Renaud's Web site recallhealing.com for information on his Recall Healing seminars given around the country. Coming soon to the www.academyCIM.com Web site will be an online course covering the content of this book.

For additional information on healing and detoxification strategies, go to www.academyCIM.com for numerous online courses given by Lee Cowden, MD, with great information covering a number of health related subjects.

listen|imagine|view|experience

AUDIO BOOK DOWNLOAD INCLUDED WITH THIS BOOK!

In your hands you hold a complete digital entertainment package. In addition to the paper version, you receive a free download of the audio version of this book. Simply use the code listed below when visiting our website. Once downloaded to your computer, you can listen to the book through your computer s speakers, burn it to an audio CD or save the file to your portable music device (such as Apple s popular iPod) and listen on the go!

How to get your free audio book digital download:

1. Visit www.tatepublishing.com and click on the e|LIVE logo on the home page.
2. Enter the following coupon code:
   9e34-3814-8dbc-2431-7dcb-ee04-b2c0-f889
3. Download the audio book from your e|LIVE digital locker and begin enjoying your new digital enter-tainment package today!